after
the first
six weeks

Also by Midwife Cath

The First Six Weeks

after the first six weeks

The tried-and-tested guide that shows you how to have
a happy, healthy and restful first year with your baby

Midwife Cath

Foreword by Dr David Sheffield, MBBS,
BMedSci, FRACP, PhD

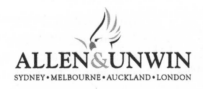

ALLEN&UNWIN
SYDNEY • MELBOURNE • AUCKLAND • LONDON

First published in 2018

Allen & Unwin
83 Alexander Street
Crows Nest NSW 2065
Australia
Phone: (61 2) 8425 0100
Email: info@allenandunwin.com
Web: www.allenandunwin.com

 A catalogue record for this
book is available from the
National Library of Australia

ISBN 978 1 76063 211 3

Illustrated by Phillip Marsden
Internal design by Bookhouse, Sydney
Index by Puddingburn Publishing Services Pty Ltd
Set in 12.5/18.8 pt Fairfield LT Std by Bookhouse, Sydney
Printed and bound in Australia by Griffin Press

10 9 8 7 6 5 4 3 2

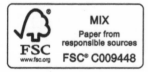

The paper in this book is FSC® certified.
FSC® promotes environmentally responsible,
socially beneficial and economically viable
management of the world's forests.

To Lachlan and Bella

Author's note

In this book I use 'he' when referring to a baby because my own baby was a boy. I also refer to babies as 'he' because so many new parents do not want to know the sex of their child (and I know) so I have trained myself to say 'he'. No offence is intended to baby girls!

There are also many types of families, and I recognise that many people parent alone. Then there are families with same-sex parents or who live within an extended family. Please read this book by adapting it as necessary to your situation. I am aware of the different family structures, and the challenges unique to each.

Foreword by Dr David Sheffield

MBBS, BMedSci, FRACP, PhD

We live in an age where information has never been easier to access and parents are confronted by abundant health information about strategies and solutions for raising their child. However, the curse of this information availability lies in its all-encompassing nature; plagued by unfiltered reproduction and regurgitation, skewed by academic sensationalism and distorted by ideological agendas. This is why I am so pleased that Cathryn Curtin has undertaken to write her second book.

I have seen firsthand how her experienced approach makes a tangible difference to the welfare of both children and their families, across multiple generations. In the fog of parenting, her methodology and timely expert support offers a beacon of considered advice that inspires confidence.

Cath is eminently qualified to provide the information contained within these pages. She has managed a birthing suite, coordinated a maternal and child health network, worked with countless practitioners and assisted thousands of parents and children in her private practice of postnatal health care. The advice Cath provides exists as a result of dedicated reflection upon her exhaustive clinical experiences. She offers practical solutions to what can seem insurmountable dilemmas unique to parents, always with the priority to enhance the relationship between parents and child, to explain what is normal and healthy and to prevent illness.

The information contained herein is a welcome antidote to the digital inaccuracies and generic information that abounds. I am confident that motivated parents will find this book invaluable and will be as grateful as I am that Cath has made the fruits of her labour—and that of so many others—available to enrich their experience over the first year of their child's life.

They say it takes a village to raise a child. We are lucky to have Midwife Cath in our global village.

Contents

Introduction

This book, a follow-up to *The First Six Weeks* (TFSW), is a comprehensive guidebook for parents, providing a roadmap to 'what's next'—starting at six weeks, a major milestone, and taking you through to the end of the first 12 months. More growth and development takes place in this first year than in any other year of your child's life, and this book will help you navigate the rest of this important first year with confidence, understand this next critical stage of your child's development and be the best parent you can be.

In *After the First Six Weeks* I discuss the joys and challenges of your child's first 12 months, focusing on such issues as breast and bottle feeding; the introduction of solids; sleep; growth and development; the importance of play; safety; and the bath, bottle and bed (BBB) routine and how it evolves over these 12 months. There's also a lot of other important information that you probably don't know you don't know!

Some of the key practices I described in detail in the first book, such as the BBB routine, will need to be adjusted to suit your baby's age, weight and stage of development, so now and then I will direct you to where you can find the detailed description and explanation of a method in *TFSW*. In this book, the goal is to fine-tune these methods, based on the age of your baby and his stage of development.

After I wrote *TFSW*, many thankful parents told me they had their baby in a perfect routine—the BBB routine—but were unsure what to do after six weeks. What happens on week seven? When could they bring back bath time? When should the dream feed stop? This book sets out to answer those questions, taking you through to your child's first birthday.

Working with pregnant women, helping babies come into the world and guiding their parents in the early years of their children's lives has been my life's work. I've worked in hospitals; in maternal and child health; with obstetricians in private practice; and today I run my own private consultancy, working with parents, in person, over the phone and over Skype—from pregnancy through to the first four years of their child's life.

I feel extremely fortunate to have always worked in a field I love. I have cared for pregnant women who are 14 years to 60 years and over, and I can say it remains a privilege to be allowed into the lives of so many families. It is incredible to be present at a birth—it is always special to see the reaction of the parents when they meet their new baby. Ten thousand babies later and counting, I can say I've seen it all, though I never get tired of seeing babies born. A new life coming into the world is something really special.

Parenting itself can come as a shock to new parents—the amount of feeding and also the difficulties that arise are challenging, such as dealing with a baby that constantly cries or cannot settle overnight, as well as coping with sleep deprivation and often conflicting advice from professionals.

It's hard to feel confident that you are doing a good job with your baby—anxiety catches us all unawares. The bubble of welcoming a newborn can feel so euphoric, and then the love for your baby deepens along with the responsibility of being a mother. It's overwhelming—a secret that can't be fully shared until you experience it. Welcome to the best club in the world! It takes time for you and your baby to settle down, so be kind to yourself, and please don't start comparing your baby to others in your mother's group or even to your other children. A new baby is a huge change to your life, your body, your self-esteem and your way of thinking. Be patient, and try to avoid consulting Dr Google.

Writing *TFSW* was an amazing experience and, after the book was published, I came into contact with so many people grateful for my common-sense approach to parenting. I was also contacted by a lot of women who were grateful that I discussed the issue of mixed feeding. I was aware of the pressure on new mothers within the community to exclusively breastfeed, but I wasn't sure just how deep it ran. It often starts in the hospital, with staff who are anti-formula and put pressure on mothers, making them feel guilty if they give their baby formula, and unsure of what to do when a new baby is hungry and crying non-stop. I discuss this issue in more detail on pages 29–30 and 111–13.

My mantra is these three words—food, love, warmth. As a parent, I believe if you go by these three words, you can't go wrong. It's simple. Keep those words in your mind. Keep saying them to yourself when you're worrying about your baby. Is your baby fed? Is he loved? Is he secure and warm, close to you?

Always talk to your baby—from birth, talking to your baby is crucial. I cannot stress enough the importance of beginning in these early days the lifetime practice of talking to your child. Don't be afraid of holding your baby and telling him what you're doing. This talk with your child will continue for the rest of your life, day after day, year after year, and become the 'voice' inside your child's head. It's important to pay attention to how you speak to your child, from day one. What is the voice your child is going to carry with him as he goes through life? Negative? Condescending? Critical? Angry? Or the voice of unconditional love and support, cultivating a sense of worthiness? Negative talk can easily become the norm and, before you know it, you have a child at two or three repeating negative talk back to you.

Always talk to your baby, especially when you are doing night feeds. Many years ago, a young mother came to me after her baby had passed away from sudden infant death syndrome (SIDS). A health professional had told her not to talk to her baby or have eye contact with him overnight; some professionals still tell mothers not to talk to their babies overnight.

This young mother was grief-stricken and heartbroken because the last time she saw her baby she turned him away and didn't talk to him. I have never forgotten her—and that's why I always encourage parents to look at their baby and talk to him day and night—especially at night. It's okay—he is your baby and you are allowed to kiss him, talk to him, love him. Those nights of early parenting pass quickly, so never let one go by without telling your baby who you are, and that you love him.

I have some 'golden rules' that you will find helpful to remember—keep this list on your fridge!

- You cannot overfeed a baby.
- You *can* underfeed a baby.
- Breast milk or formula is the main source of food for the baby's first 12 months.
- Healthy, well babies who are born at term cry for two reasons—hunger and discomfort. The discomfort is usually associated with gastric reflux.

- Babies need to be at least 7 to 8 kilograms to have the capacity to sleep a good stretch overnight.
- Babies need to be old enough to have the capacity to sleep well overnight.
- A newborn baby won't self-settle; he needs to feed to sleep.

So many women tell me, 'No one told me it would be this hard.' Even for those that are forwarned, it's really hard to imagine how much life will change until your baby arrives. I want this book to be a positive guide for you in these first twelve months as a parent. I want to continue to be the positive voice in your head. And when the first birthday arrives, plan a big celebration for surviving this first difficult but amazing year!

PART 1
BECOMING PARENTS

1

Safety in the home

Babies need constant supervision. Many injuries can occur within the home and our little children are at the greatest risk. The most common causes of injury to young children are burns, finger jams, falls, poisoning and near-drowning. Most of these are predictable and preventable.

Keep an eye on your baby's older sibling(s)

Be careful when toddlers hold your baby as they quickly lose attention. I have seen a toddler drop a baby on the floor and just walk off. That's the way toddlers think—it's all about them. They mean no harm, so don't reprimand your child. But if your toddler wants to hold your baby, sit with him, helping him hold the baby, and then after a few minutes say that's enough. Give the toddler some boundaries—a beginning and an end to the session.

My baby was only four weeks old when I introduced him to my girlfriends and their young children. I put baby George to sleep upstairs as there were lots of toddlers and I didn't want him to be disturbed by them. We were having lunch when a three-year-old toddler, Lily, arrived carrying George! To this day I do not know how she got him out of the cot and down the stairs, maybe I don't want to know. What I do know is that from then on, I always had my eyes on George if there were other children around.

— SARAH

First aid training

I think it's vital for all parents of babies and young children to do a first aid course. I hope you never need it but if you do, your knowledge and expertise will come in handy. There are companies that train new parents in paediatric resuscitation. Do your research to ensure that the educators conducting the training have a medical background and then, ideally, attend first aid training before your first baby is born.

Keep a fully stocked first aid kit in your house, and another one in the car, but make sure they're both out of reach of small children. For parents who have previously done a first aid course, I would advise them to do a refresher course prior to the birth of the baby. We can forget quickly. You never know when you'll need it!

Baby-proofing your home

When I studied maternal and child health at university, I can remember a teacher telling us the best way to safety-proof a house for a baby was to get down on our hands and knees and crawl around to see what a baby could see. I thought this was a stupid idea but I was young and I didn't have a child then. When I did have my son, I began to understand what she was talking about. I got down onto my hands and knees and had a good look around to check for potential problems for a moving baby. So here we go—everyone on your hands and knees, let's check the house!

A baby can put anything in his mouth—a coin, a battery, a small toy, a bit of food or even a piece of fluff may be on the floor and they are all potentially choking hazards. Also look out for curtain and blind cords that reach the floor (the baby can get caught in them) and pet food bowls (the baby might think the pet food looks appetising). He might be rolling around on the floor from the age of 15 weeks so it's best to get things done before there are any accidents or dramas. Prevention far outweighs the cure! For example, his fingers can get caught in cupboard drawers and doors; he can choke on nuts and other hard foods, be suffocated by plastic bags and even cot sheets or doonas, be poisoned by cleaning products that aren't stored in locked cupboards, be bitten by animals and he can drown if unsupervised near a swimming pool. If your house has stairs, install safety gates at both the top and bottom.

The baby's room

Safety in the home starts with a safe sleeping environment. It's really important to position both the change table and the cot away from any long curtain or blind cords that your baby can grab. Cords are a strangling risk for babies and young children.

Have everything you need for the change table within your reach so you never have to leave the baby alone on the table. Even before the birth, make sure you have all the nappies, cotton balls, biodegradable baby wipes, singlets, sets of clothes, various creams and nappy rash powder close by in a secure drawer on the change table.

Never give your child a tube of cream to play with while you're changing him. I've seen lots of mothers hand the baby a tube of cream they're going to use on his bottom to keep their baby occupied. He can easily bite on the tube and swallow the contents. Keep a small rattle or toy nearby to use when you're changing your baby, because as he gets older he will move, turn, squirm and protest while you do so, and a toy will help quieten him.

Never, ever leave a baby alone on a change table—even for a second. A baby can squirm and fall off the table in the time it takes you to turn around or bend down to pick something up off the floor! I know it sounds ridiculous, but they can. If your eyes are off your baby, keep your hands on your baby. I've heard so many stories from parents who said, 'I only turned around for a second or two . . .' Don't risk it. If you have to turn around, hold onto your baby's leg and then do what you need to do, but if you have to leave the room, don't leave him alone on the bed or the change table—either take him with you, or pop him on the floor or in his cot.

The baby's cot must meet Australian standards to ensure your baby's safety. If you have a cot on loan from a friend, I would encourage you to buy a new mattress that is firm and fits adequately into the cot. A poorly fitted mattress can be dangerous as a baby can slip down between the mattress and the cot. Put a mattress protector under a clean fitted sheet—nothing else should be in the cot.

Test any nightlights and lamps but remember, it isn't necessary to have a light on all night in your baby's room.

Make sure all power points are covered at all times to prevent your moving child poking anything into the socket.

Safe sleeping for babies

Red Nose provides safe sleeping guidelines to reduce the incidence of fatal sleeping accidents in Australia. It is advised that all parents adhere to the following guidelines:

- Sleep your baby on his back from birth, not on his tummy or side.
- Sleep your baby with his face and head uncovered and free from bedding, pillows and toys.
- Avoid exposing your baby to tobacco smoke before birth and after.
- Provide a safe sleeping environment with safe furniture and bedding: this means no quilts, doonas, duvets or pillows in the cot.
- Sleep your baby in his own safe sleeping place in the same room as you for the first six to 12 months.
- Breastfeed if you can.

The bathroom

Once your baby starts moving, he may follow you when you go to the bathroom! When you are home alone and need to go to the toilet, or want to have a shower, place your baby in a safe place, like his cot, or in a playpen if you have one. It will only be for a few minutes—a short time and you deserve to have a relaxing shower by yourself!

Hand sanitiser is used in most bathrooms these days and is usually carried in nappy bags. I see parents applying it to baby's and toddler's hands—toddlers are even capable of 'pumping' the disinfectant onto their own hands! I applaud parents for being careful with cross-contamination, but I feel it has gone to the extreme. Hand sanitiser contains between 60 and 95 per cent ethanol or isopropyl alcohol, and if taken orally could be fatal to a young child. It can also cause eye pain, as the baby or toddler may rub his eyes with his hand, still wet with sanitiser, causing irritation and discomfort. Sanitiser should be strictly supervised by parents to prevent any harm, minor or major, to the little ones. In the bathroom at home, good old soap and water is as effective as any sanitiser. When out of the house, unscented baby wipes are safer and preferable to wipe the hands and face of a baby or toddler.

Before you have the baby, be prepared and put childproof locks on bathroom cupboards so you can keep dangerous appliances and toiletries well out of baby's reach. These days there's a huge range to choose from and they're cheap and easy to install.

These include:

- medicine, tablets, lotions, creams, make-up, perfume and detergents

- scissors, razor blades, tweezers, toothbrushes, hair dryers, shavers and heaters
- liquid hand soaps and hand sanitisers.

Children can drown in very small amounts of water, so always keep the toilet seat down. Walk around your house and try to look at it from a baby's perspective.

When you bath your baby in a big bath, prevent him from slipping by placing a non-slip mat underneath him. Babies love to jump and move around in the bath so you must hold him at all times. Never leave a baby or small child alone in the bath as accidents happen and they happen quickly.

The living area

It's important to ensure that the TV is secure, ideally bolted to the wall, as children can pull them down on top of themselves, oblivious to the dangers of pulling on the TV. Install childproof locks on all cupboards, drawers and anything else your baby can access in the living area, and remove any objects, such as vases, from table- and cupboard tops.

The kitchen

A kitchen can be a dangerous place and is really not safe for young children. It's a good idea to keep a fire blanket handy at all times in case of an accident on the stove, and also to install child safety locks on all the cupboards and drawers.

If you're having friends over for a meal or afternoon tea, think twice before laying the table with a tablecloth. A baby can tug on the tablecloth and pull down hot drinks and crockery on top of himself, risking injury and severe burns.

When you are drinking a hot drink, it's best to either put the baby down into the pram or cot or hand your baby to someone else. When a baby sees a coffee mug/tea cup, he is likely to instinctively grab for it (they are so strong) and pull it towards himself. Before you know it, the baby may have tipped a hot drink over himself. Scalds are terrible burns and are preventable.

When your baby is old enough to sit up in a highchair, look at one that has the Australian Standards seal of approval. Use the built-in harness on your baby every time he sits in the highchair—he will not only get used to the harness but eventually expect to have the harness on when he is in the highchair. If you start from day 1, it will become a habit, not only for you but also for your baby. But don't rely on the highchair to keep him safe if you need to leave the room—I've seen injured babies after they've rocked the highchair so vigorously, they made it fall over!

Cars

When you put a baby or a toddler in a hot car, the car seat can be very hot, too, causing the baby's temperature to rise very quickly. On a sunny day, put your car's air-conditioner on for at least five minutes before you take the baby out of the house. According to Kidsafe Victoria, 'The temperature inside a parked car during the Australian summer can be 20 to 30 degrees hotter than the outside temperature. On a 29-degree Celsius day a car can reach 44 degrees in just 10 minutes and a deadly 60 degrees in 20 minutes. Leaving the window down a few centimetres does little.'

Never leave your child alone in the car, even while you run back into the house to fetch something you've forgotten, or dash into a service station to pay for petrol. For one thing, opportunistic car thieves have been known to hop into cars and drive off with children in the back seat. This happened to my sister, so I know only too well how easily it can happen.

One of the biggest causes of accidental death of children is cars reversing. Even if your car has a reversing camera that shows what's behind the car when you reverse, you should never rely on it alone—always check to see that children are in the car with you or safely in the house or supervised by adults before reversing out of a garage or driveway.

Car restraints

When leaving the hospital, you are required by law to place your baby in a safe, suitable and approved car restraint that faces the back of the car. The approved car restraint for the baby will have an appropriate sticker saying that it complies with the Australian and New Zealand Standards. Did you know it's actually illegal to use car restraints that have been purchased overseas?

You must have the car restraint fitted properly by a reputable tradesman, such as one from an official motoring association—the RACV or equivalent in your state. Even when you're travelling in a taxi or Uber, you must have the baby in an approved car seat at all times, so if you're away from home and your own car, have a car seat and its attachments available to enable you to assemble it in someone else's car.

Never allow your child to stand up in the back seat or sit on anyone's lap—it is both dangerous and illegal.

Prams

Ensure you buy a pram that conforms to Australian Standards, and has strong safety straps to fasten the baby safely and securely. These days you can buy convertible prams that adjust to a baby's age and stage of development. Try out different types in the shop—a pram should be the right height for you so you can walk comfortably with it, and have enough room for baby's nappy bag and small amounts of shopping. Also make sure you're able to get it in and out of your car quickly and easily.

Why you shouldn't cover the pram

Please don't put a muslin wrap over the pram. Your baby needs to see your face as well as look around. Covering the pram disengages a baby from the outside world; it does *not* encourage him to go to sleep.

It can also be very hot and stuffy underneath a muslin wrap. Sometimes I even see a blanket over a baby's pram. In Australia we try to keep our babies out of the sun, but studies conducted in Sweden showed that covering a pram caused the inside temperature to reach 22 degrees. With a muslin wrap over the pram for 30 minutes, the heat rose to 34 degrees. After an hour it had risen to 37 degrees. Can you imagine the heat inside the pram if it was tested in Australian heat? This would put babies at a greater danger of heatstroke and other health risks such as SIDS.

So, if you go walking, let the baby play in the pram and enjoy the fresh air. If he's still young enough to be lying down in the pram, facing you, talk to him.

Sun safety tips

Sun safety is something we Australians need to live with. Your child will need to use sunscreen all his life to protect him from the harsh Australian sun; in fact, babies under six months should not be exposed to the sun at all. Whenever you're outside with your baby, keep him dressed in a hat and in the shade as much as possible. If there are reflective surfaces, such as mirrors or glass-topped tables around, he can still get burned, so cover him all over.

Between 10 am and 4 pm, when the sun's rays are the hottest, keep your baby inside to prevent sunburn and heat-stroke. And in the car, install a window shade to protect the baby from the sun, as ultraviolet radiation can filter through the windows.

Sunscreen

Babies' skin is different from adult skin—underneath the top layer, it is very fragile and sensitive. Most sunscreens are *not* recommended for babies under six months because the skin can potentially absorb more chemicals, and babies can often be allergic or sensitive to sunscreen. Your baby's skin is so sensitive and precious; it is best to keep him indoors during the early months of his life. For older children, apply an even, thick layer of creamy SPF 50+ sunscreen (do not use an aerosol spray), to their exposed skin every two hours. Pay particular attention to the back of the neck, the ears, face, legs, feet and even the soles of the feet. Then reapply it after they've been in the water, first drying their skin with a towel. It is important to note that you should not leave sunscreen in the car as heat may deactivate the chemicals and make the sunscreen ineffective.

Drowning prevention

You must always supervise children around water—whether it's a swimming pool, a dam, a paddling pool or a bath. By all means use flotation devices, but don't treat them as life-saving devices. Always stay with your child. Always.

Any body of water on your property—even if it's a small pond—should be fenced. Each state has guidelines for the height of mandatory fences and gates around pools, but you also need to check that children can't climb fences by pushing a chair over or jumping from a tree branch overhanging the pool. You must always check that the gate to the pool is locked and in good condition. Never let children swim alone. An adult must be with them, supervising at all times.

As soon as he's old enough, have your child taught to swim by a qualified swim instructor and, as I've already recommended, learn CPR from an accredited professional.

2

Caring for your baby

Your baby needs you, and you will spend many hours feeding him, changing his nappy and just staring at him. Many women say they are unprepared for the round-the-clock care a baby requires. It is impossible to prepare anyone for early parenting. What we can do is provide an extended village to first-time parents within the community. They need support from maternal and child health (MCH) nurses to guide and educate them about the health and development of their new baby, as well as support in the home from family and friends.

Feeding your baby

Some babies are born little, some babies are born big, but all babies are hungry. They need to be fed. You cannot overfeed a baby but you can *underfeed* a baby. I see far too many babies who have been underfed and diagnosed with colic, reflux and allergies, with professionals telling their mothers they have 'an incorrect latch'. These babies are *so* hungry. Make sure you feed your baby enough.

> I went to the maternal and child health nurse so happy and proud of my baby as I thought I was doing a great job. My baby was eight weeks old, exclusively breastfed; she was sleeping for six hours after the 10 o'clock bath and I was feeling really well. She had put on 300 grams in a week and I was told, 'You're overfeeding her, you need to cut back on your feeds.' I was devastated. Instantly I felt like a bad mother. I cried all the way home and my husband reminded me that we have a healthy baby who sleeps and feeds well. Looking back now I can see how silly the nurse's comment was, but I was feeling so vulnerable as a new mum; I thought I was going to be praised for breastfeeding well and having a baby who slept.
>
> — ANNIE

Back in the days when women stayed in hospital for ten to fourteen days, midwives understood and trusted the process of how women's bodies changed as the milk slowly came in over days three, four and five. The babies were sleepy and were offered formula overnight so the mothers could rest and recover from the birth. We never let babies cry with hunger, and we made sure they were fed as we waited for the mother's milk to come in. These babies rarely lost 10 per cent of their birth weight as they do now, and they were not screaming with hunger. We would sit with the new mums for hours, teaching them about breastfeeding, and we didn't rush them out of hospital.

These days midwives are well trained and have good intent but unfortunately they only see new mothers for three to four days post-natally in the hospital. Their advice is correct for those few days but not appropriate as the baby grows, wakes up, and changes his feeding and sleeping patterns. And believe me, a baby who is four, six, seven, eight weeks old is a very different baby from one who is one, two or three weeks old. My aim is successful long-term breastfeeding, and we must teach new mums in the early weeks to give them the confidence to continue feeding. New parents refer back to what they learnt from the hospital midwives in the few days after the birth and that's how they continue to care for their baby. I see it time and again.

Take, for example, the sleepy baby, a very common sight in the postnatal ward in the first few days. Midwives encourage parents to make sure their baby is awake and uncomfortable during feeding so he will suck properly: they suggest undressing the baby and unwrapping him to keep him cold, flicking him on the toes, blowing in his face, and putting a cold face washer on his body.

Mother Nature does not want babies to be cold and fearful when feeding at the breast. It just doesn't make sense. To me it seems crazy that a midwife would tell a new mum to unwrap and undress their baby to make them cold and uncomfortable so they feed! When I explain the alternative to parents, they inevitably tell me that it never made sense to them either, but as they were being told by a professional, they thought it must be right. When you are a new parent and on your own in hospital, you're vulnerable, and when you have a professional telling you to undress your sleepy baby, blow in his face and flick his feet to encourage him to feed, you assume you are doing the right thing, and you do it.

New parents really are the easiest of all patients to care for because they want to do the right thing for their baby, even if what they're being told goes against their gut instincts. I saw one new mother in my private consulting room with her two-week-old baby who was not sleeping overnight at all. When the mother arrived, the baby was only in a singlet and light, short-sleeved onesie—not wrapped. I explained to the mum that dressing and wrapping the baby would be the best thing to do, as this would not only keep the baby warm but help the baby feel more secure.

Once we did that, the baby fed on both breasts and went to sleep. The mother said she had never seen her do so. There were lots of tears, shame, sadness and frustration. She told me she knew what was right, but had to believe what she had been told in hospital. The baby continued to feed well after being dressed and wrapped, and her mother continued to breastfeed for twelve months.

The importance of having informed options before the birth

We all hear about birth plans and parents try to make informed choices about how they want their baby to enter the world; however, in many cases, things don't always go to plan. This is the same for feeding your newborn. As a nurse, midwife and MCH health nurse with more than 40 years' experience, I often comfort and advise distressed parents about what to do when breastfeeding doesn't initially work. For some women, all the pieces of the puzzle come together and their newborn can feed from their breasts within minutes of their birth. But for many others, their milk doesn't come through quickly enough, they suffer from mastitis, or sore and cracked nipples, and their babies may not attach properly—the list goes on. It comes to many women as a surprise when they discover that breastfeeding is not always that easy.

I always tell my clients to come prepared with informed options. For example, what happens if your baby is premature or sick? What if your baby is losing weight or crying all the time because he is still hungry? When does your baby need formula? Why do you have to sign a form to give your baby formula?

New parents pick up so much inconsistent information through social media, published articles, friends, family and books . . . The aim of an informed feeding plan is to eliminate any confusion and conflicting advice and come to hospital knowledgeable and ready. Trying to make decisions when you have just had your baby and are sleep deprived as well as possibly medicated and in pain is extremely difficult.

Creating a plan before the baby is born—at 34 to 36 weeks—empowers parents and allows them to feel in control and prepared for the unpredictably of birth and what comes soon after.

Nothing can truly prepare you for motherhood. The books I read were a great guide on what to expect and what I could do for each stage, but nothing can truly connect you with the emotions you will feel when that child is placed in your arms for the first time.

I thought breastfeeding would come so naturally to me. I knew my mum wasn't able to breastfeed me, but I knew I would have a good supply of milk as I had been waking up in the morning from around 28 to 29 weeks in my pregnancy with my pyjama top and bed sheets wet from leaking.

Unfortunately, that was no indication of how I would find breastfeeding.

My daughter Sienna weighed 3.1 kilograms at birth and just wouldn't latch on, even with the aid of a nipple shield. Each feed, the midwives from the hospital would manually express me and feed my daughter via a syringe, then top her up with some formula.

I remember one midwife manually expressing me so hard with her hands that when I went to sleep that night, I felt as if my breasts were on fire. I wanted what was best for Sienna but the pain was excruciating.

The minute we were told when I would be discharged, I phoned Cath and asked if we could see her.

As soon as we sat down with Cath, everything changed. I'll never forget her telling me we were starting with Plan A and, if need be, we would go right up to Plan Z! That comment immediately made me think, I can do this! It'll be fine.

The first plan was to express what I could and offer it through a bottle, topping up with formula if need be. It wasn't long till we noticed our once small daughter starting to have some noticeably fuller cheeks! The next step was to try to attach Sienna at feeds for a few minutes on each side and express what I could in between, topping up with formula if need be. This seemed to work, which meant we were slowly getting closer to being able to breastfeed with ease. We then decided we would breastfeed at every meal and stop expressing. Unfortunately, this is where things changed, Sienna did not want to attach for long enough to get a good feed, and in one instance held her breath in protest at being breastfed.

My supply changed dramatically. I went from not being able to breastfeed without the other side leaking everywhere to barely leaking at all, including during the night. It was around four weeks that Cath and I discussed feeding Sienna on formula only. Sienna was becoming stressed when I attempted to breastfeed, and I was not enjoying my time with her because I was becoming stressed at every feed, knowing it would be a battle to have her latch on, and stay latched on.

We had a couple of successful feeds but not enough. While I was disappointed that I wasn't able to breastfeed, especially when I knew I had such a good supply to start with, I ended up with the result I wanted from the moment I found out I was pregnant—a healthy, happy and well-fed baby.

While all these plans were being tried and tested, we were lucky enough to have the support of my mum every day, ensuring the house was kept clean and we had a good meal each night. This allowed us to focus solely on Sienna and getting her to feed without worrying about anything else. It also allowed us to bond with Sienna in those very important first weeks of her life.

Cath supported us, no matter what our concerns were. I was confused and stressed after my first visit to the maternal health care nurse. She told me that my daughter had a tongue-tie, lip-tie (which she didn't) and a hernia in her stomach which, if it grew, would need to be operated on. Sienna's paediatrician examined her and advised us that she did not have a hernia at all.

We will be forever grateful for the knowledge and friendship we received from Cath.

— ROSIE

Breastfeeding

Your baby has an innate, primitive will to suck and live, and to live he must suck your milk. Here's a refresher on breastfeeding, which is covered in greater detail in *TFSW*.

First of all, I wrap babies for all feeds (see 'Cath's Wrap', page 34). To breastfeed your baby in comfort I suggest you follow these pointers: hold the baby, on his side facing you across your chest with his ear in the crook of your elbow. If you are feeding from the left breast, place him in your left

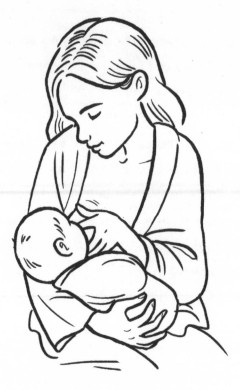

Always wrap your baby when feeding

arm. Let him suck the nipple in by himself, rolling him into your breast with the arm that is holding him.

Hold your breast with your right hand in the peace sign: three fingers below the nipple and one above, very gently pressing your breast to help your nipple face upwards so the baby's mouth can find the nipple. You do not need to get all the areola in. Some women have large areolas and it is impossible for the baby to have all this in his mouth. It's black and white—if your baby is sucking your nipple, he is ON the breast and sucking well!

Do not express any milk—let your baby do the work. He is the best pump! Do not force him on by hand or let anyone else hold his head and force him onto your breast. And don't keep taking your baby on and off the breast, as this will damage your nipple.

If your baby has not passed urine in 12 hours and is losing weight, give him some formula as some free kilojoules. This will prevent the baby from losing too much weight and resulting in you having a crying and distressed baby. Both you and your baby will feel better. Don't worry—your breasts will continue to fill, you will lactate, you will continue to breastfeed, plus your baby will gain weight! It makes sense, doesn't it?

Do not give a hungry baby a dummy. The dummy has no kilojoules and the baby needs food—milk.

Engorged breasts and sore nipples

If your breasts are engorged with milk, do not massage them at any time or let anyone else touch them. Your breasts are inflamed and working very hard. Compare your lactating breasts to a broken and swollen ankle—you would not massage it as it would cause harm (and pain) to the tissue, and the same applies to your breasts. Leave them alone.

Take oral anti-inflammatory tablets and paracetamol for sore breasts to help with the inflammation and put only breast milk on your nipples. Do not use any creams, potions or lotions as these can lead to infection ascending through your nipples to your breasts and can cause mastitis (see page 90).

If there is not enough milk coming out of your engorged breasts, have the baby suck for a small amount of time (5 minutes each side only) then offer your baby a drink of formula while you wait for your breasts to settle. It will take a few days, but they will settle; the breasts will become soft and the baby will be able to suck a lot easier from the breast. You just need to be patient. Do *not* express or pump your breasts—it will only make them sore and hard, and will increase your risk of mastitis. Give your body time to recover, then let your baby do the work by sucking at the breast.

Apply cold cabbage leaves to your breasts, after you have washed the leaves and put them in the freezer to cool. When the cabbage leaves warm up, replace with more cold leaves. You won't eat cabbage again for some time! Wear a firm bra that supports your breasts well and keep up your medication.

Feed your baby frequently. Never use water, or sugar and water—just breast milk and/or formula for babies younger than twelve months. If your baby is still hungry, give him some formula. He will gain weight faster and you will breastfeed for longer.

If your breasts are so engorged that your nipples have flattened, use a nipple shield (see page 88) to add length to your nipples. When your breasts have settled, the baby will reattach to your nipple again to suck.

If you have damaged, sore and/or cracked nipples, do *not* take the baby off the breast. Put on a nipple shield to help your nipples heal within 24 to 48 hours. The wonderful healing power of the breast milk pooling within the shield will help your nipple recover quickly.

Bottle-feeding

There are many reasons why some babies need to be fed formula. Some women simply can't breastfeed at all, or have personal reasons for not breastfeeding, while others have trouble producing enough milk to sustain a healthy weight in their baby. Premature babies, who are born with a limited reflex to suck, may need a bottle in the early days to ensure good and consistent weight gain.

I am a strong advocate for breastfeeding and I encourage women to breastfeed long term, but I also respect and support the right of each woman to make her own choice. It's the parenting that's important, as well as the input of the partner and loving and caring for the baby—and it's futile to make a mother feel guilty if she can't or won't breastfeed.

There's no scientific evidence that your baby will not take a nipple after he's given a bottle, and having a bottle will not confuse your baby or decrease your breast milk. I have looked after thousands of babies that feed successfully off both—they breastfeed and take one or more bottles during the day. Babies are really smart. Babies who only use a bottle at some feeds, as in my BBB routine, will not experience nipple confusion when breastfeeding. Babies never refuse the breast, but they will refuse a bottle if they have not been given a bottle within the first four to six weeks. Often they will continue to refuse a bottle completely, which can be a huge problem if the mother is ill, in hospital, weaning the baby or going back to work. Believe me, if you want your baby to take a bottle long term you must offer either formula or expressed milk to him in a bottle within the first weeks after birth.

If your baby used formula while in hospital, you'll probably continue with the same one. If, on the other hand, your baby started formula-feeding after hospital, you'll receive recommendations from your health professionals. If your child experiences any reaction to a formula recommended by an MCH nurse or paediatrician, you can change the formula. But don't change it without medical advice.

What you'll need

To bottle-feed a baby, you'll need:

- a reliable electric steriliser
- six to eight bottles

- a bottle-cleaner for washing the bottles and teats properly after each use and before sterilising
- a large plastic container that can be used to hold all the sterilised bottles in the fridge, which will reduce the risk of any bacteria growing in the bottles.

If you plan to only bottle-feed or your baby needs some extra formula top-ups, I suggest you buy a formula machine that warms the water to create the perfect baby bottle with the push of one button. They are fabulous and save so much time.

How to bottle-feed a baby

Wrap the baby so he feels secure, then cradle him in your left arm while holding the bottle at a 45-degree angle in your right hand. Place the teat near the baby's mouth and as he opens it gently allow the baby to suck the teat in. Make sure the teat is full of milk during feeding so he doesn't take in air.

If milk is dribbling out the side of his mouth, check that the lid on the bottle has been firmly screwed on. Don't worry too much if your baby gulps while he is bottle-feeding; he will only drink as much as he can cope with. Sometimes a baby will put his tongue on his top palate, preventing him from feeding properly, so check that his tongue is down when you put the teat in his mouth.

If you wish to offer your baby a bottle while breastfeeding, offer it in the first few weeks after birth. How much to give

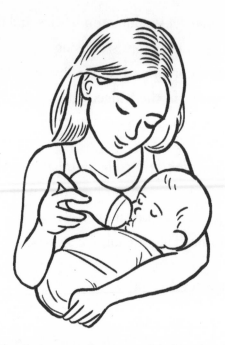

Hold the bottle at a 45-degree angle when bottle-feeding
and keep your baby wrapped

a baby depends on his age, weight and maturity, so consult your paediatrician or MCH nurse.

How to prepare formula

For convenience, I have repeated my instructions from *TFSW*, page 103.

- Wash a glass jug in hot soapy water and rinse with hot water from the tap.

- Stand the jug in the sink and fill it with just boiled water.
- Wash and sterilise a whisk by placing a clean one in the boiled water in the glass jug. Leave the whisk in the jug for three minutes, then drain.
- Boil the kettle again. Pour the water out of the jug and refill it with the correct amount of boiling water, then add the correct number of scoops of formula.
- Put the whisk in the formula and thoroughly mix the powder and water together. Place a lid on the jug and refrigerate immediately.
- Use the formula for 24 hours only and discard any unused formula.
- Each time you need to feed the baby, pour the selected amount of formula into a sterilised bottle and heat it by using a bottle warmer or standing the bottle in a mug of hot water.
- Always shake the bottle before you give it to the baby to ensure that the formula is the correct temperature. Any unused formula in each bottle must be thrown out.

Cath's Wrap

When he was in utero, your baby was firmly contained by a strong wall of muscle, but once he was born, his primitive reflexes—such as the Moro or startle reflex, which makes him throw his arms out as if he's trying to grab onto something for

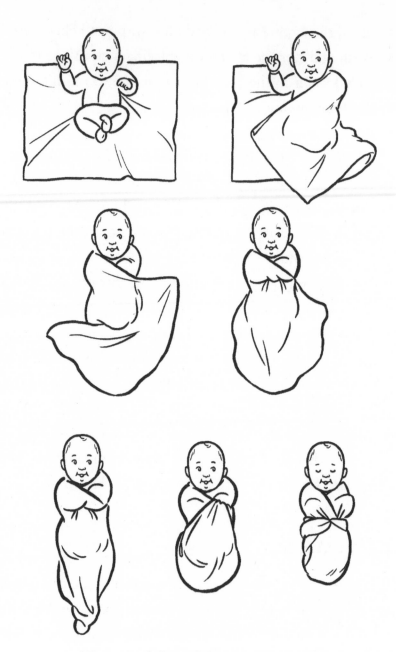

Wrap your baby with his arms bent up

fear of falling—make him feel insecure. After years of observing babies, I invented a simple, yet effective, way to wrap babies that makes them feel safe, secure and calm, helping them to feed better and sleep well. You'll need a soft, lightweight muslin wrap that is at least 1.2 x 1.4 metres to wrap your baby with his hands and arms bent up and his hips able to flex. If you wrap him with his hands by his sides and his hips unable to flex, he will fight it and squirm so much you will think he is unhappy and that he 'hates the wrap'. Inevitably his hands will end up out of the wrap and scratching his face.

I recommend that you wrap your baby for all feeds and all sleep in his first six weeks, then continue to wrap him for all sleep until he is six months old. By this age the startle reflex will have settled, and you can then put him into a sleeping bag for sleep.

Wrapping also means you don't have to wrestle with those busy hands—I've even seen a dad holding the baby's hands down while the mum attempts to breastfeed. It helps to wrap when you feed and when your baby is going to sleep. (See also *TFSW*, page 138.)

My famous BBB routine

My bath, bottle and bed (BBB) routine, designed for a baby in his twelfth month of life is really very simple.

- **Bath** the baby every night at 10 pm, even if he is asleep.
- Offer a **bottle** of formula to the baby after the bath every night.
- Put him straight to **bed** after the bottle.

I encourage mums to go to bed to get some well-earned rest, plus a physical and psychological break from the baby, and leave their partners to take charge of the bath and bottle. This gives partners precious time bathing, holding, washing, dressing and feeding the baby. It becomes their gig!

Passing a few practical chores onto your partner or another member of the household will help you, and the rest of the family, enormously. If you find it hard to go to bed and relax, put on some meditation music and try to slow down your thinking. It's often hard to 'tune out' the fact that your baby is being bathed and fed by someone else. As mothers, we tend to 'hover' over our partners, as we think we can do all things associated with baby better.

As for your baby, this routine helps him to have his longest sleep in the 24-hour period after the bath. In his first few weeks he is only capable of sleeping three to four hours at the most, but, as he gains weight during weeks 3 to 6, he will sleep longer—up to six hours.

So, partners, while mum gets some rest you should bath your baby in a deep, warm bath (38°C) with no seat, so he can relax in the water (for detailed instructions on bathing

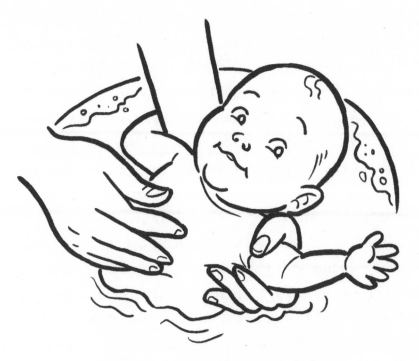

Bath your baby in a deep, warm bath

a baby, see page 44). Don't worry about using any soap or solution in the early days as his skin is very pure. Most babies will have very dry skin in the first few days after birth and this will peel off; then the baby's skin will be soft and beautiful.

When you have finished bathing the baby, take him out of the water and lay him down on a towel. He may cry when he is naked before and after the bath, so just explain to him what you are doing, and undress and dress him as soon as you can.

Once you have dried the baby, dress him for bed. Always dress the baby in his nappy, a singlet (even in hot weather), a onesie and then in Cath's Wrap (see page 33). Give him a bottle of either expressed breast milk or formula. In the early days, you can offer him up to 90 ml. Even if you think he won't take that much, prepare it anyway just in case he finishes the full bottle—you don't want to interrupt this peaceful routine by going off to the kitchen to make up another one. And remember, you can't overfeed a baby.

Until about four weeks, your baby may take up to 120 ml, depending on his birth weight—that is, a baby who was under 3 kilograms at birth may only take 50 ml, but a baby who was over 4 kilograms at birth may take 120 ml.

Once he is calm and going to sleep, place him on your shoulder and very gently massage his back. Sometimes just popping him on your shoulder will make him burp by himself. You don't have to bang has back—remember, he is only a little baby—be very gentle with him. Then put him down safely in the bassinet with a light muslin wrap over him to tuck him in. Do not put layers and layers of blankets on him as this will overheat him and is a SIDS risk. He should be dressed in a singlet and a onesie, wrapped in the muslin wrap and then a second muslin firmly tucked in around him.

If he does not go to sleep straight away and is looking for more food, pick him up and unwrap him, then give him some tummy time, some back time, then maybe some more

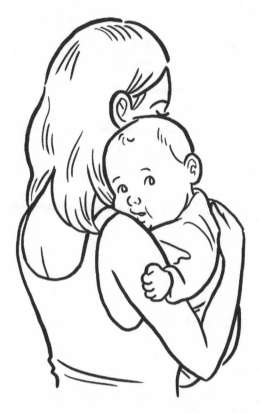

Place your baby on your shoulder and gently rub
his back to burp him

tummy time, change his nappy, rewrap him and offer him
another bottle. By this stage he should be ready for sleep, so
tuck him in and then head to bed yourself.

Babies are very squirmy and noisy at night; it helps to
put the cot on an angle, up to 45 degrees. Some babies with
reflux tend to be noisier than others.

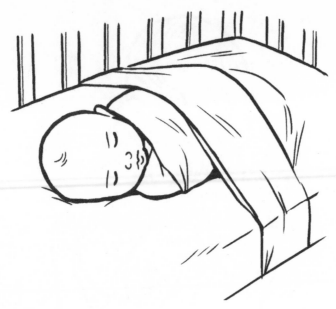

In the cot, your baby doesn't need layers of blankets

By the time your baby next wakes—probably around 2 or 3 am, the mother has enjoyed a deep sleep for up to five hours. The partner also sleeps after the BBB routine and is off duty until the morning. Women are hormonally charged to cope with getting up and feeding the baby, and cope with sleep deprivation and interruption of sleep much better than men do.

My BBB routine helps women to breastfeed longer—well over 12 months—as it gives them a basic routine to follow, a decent break from the baby and the ability to sleep for more than three hours at a time. It's all due to teamwork.

This process has been tried successfully by thousands of my patients and remains a successful routine for the first 10 to 14 weeks. The 10 pm bath won't be forever. As your baby gets older and puts on more weight, you will make bath time earlier. It's all about weight gain and the age of the baby. A newborn baby of 3 kilograms is not capable of sleeping longer than two to three hours, but with lots of food (breast milk and/or formula), he will slowly but surely start to sleep longer, after the 10 pm bath and bottle routine.

You need to be patient and consistent, and your baby will start to sleep for four to five hours, then six to seven and eight hours. It takes at least eight to nine weeks to start to make a change. Patience is the first skill we as parents need to learn. The nights you wake up to your new baby are few in the overall scheme of things, and don't last long, even though you feel so very tired.

In a couple of weeks, you will bath him at 9.30 pm, then 9 pm, and by slow increments the baby will eventually have a bath at about 6 pm, have a feed and go to bed. Then introduce the 'dream feed' at 10 pm when the baby is asleep (see page 164).

The bath time gets earlier but the bottle always stays at 10 pm as a dream feed or rollover feed. This provides 'free kilojoules' so your baby can sleep past midnight till about 4 or 5 am!

A baby can put on an *average* of 150 grams per week. Not all babies can or will gain weight at the same rate, so it's best not to start comparing your baby with other babies. We all can't be 190 centimetres tall and weigh 90 kilograms. Some babies put on up to 300 grams a week, while others put on less than 150 grams per week. This is normal for a baby who is well, in proportion, and eating and sleeping well. As long as your baby is continuing to gain weight and is well and happy, passing urine and having a poo, he is well.

When your baby is about four months old and weighs around 8 kilograms, he has the capacity to sleep longer. At this age, the baby can be bathed at 6 pm, wrapped, breastfed and put to bed around 7 pm. Then every night, until the baby is 12 months old, your partner can pick the baby up at 10 pm while he's asleep and give him a bottle-feed—this is the 'dream feed' or 'rollover feed' that gives the baby extra kilojoules to sleep through the night and continue weight gain so he will grow and sleep for longer periods. Your partner can then cuddle the baby and settle him back into his bed.

I would then expect a baby at that age and weight to wake again around 3 or 4 am for a breastfeed, and then go back to sleep till 6 to 7 am. It sounds easy but it means a lot of feeding. One bottle of formula at night will not do any harm to your breast milk, and giving your baby a bottle will not cause any 'nipple confusion'.

If your baby has reflux or any other medical condition, he will not easily fall into the sleep routine. Seek help if your baby is crying more than you think is normal.

I would like to thank you for setting me up with the most incredible foundations to start my first-time mum role. Harry is nine weeks old now, and has been sleeping nine hours overnight since six weeks, and is absolutely thriving. I feel extremely confident and relaxed, and it's because of the very simple advice you gave us. A midwife in my mother's group recently told me that I might be overfeeding Harry and that I should try to stop him when he's still going and just give him a dummy. I was fortunate enough to know that you can't overfeed a baby, and why would I, when he's a very happy and content baby? When we went home to New Zealand for Christmas I told anyone who would listen about Cath's BBB routine and absolutely swear by it.

— SARAH

When to bring the bath time back

As your baby gains weight and sleeps longer past midnight, slowly bring bath-time forward in 30-minute increments over the course of a few weeks. But there is no hurry to do this as every baby handles being bathed earlier in his own way.

Bathing your baby

Bathing your baby can be a wonderful experience for you both as it is calming and relaxing for him. Before you begin, have everything organised—the bath filled with warm water, deep enough so it comes right up to your baby's neck, and clean towels and face washers, some nappies, a clean outfit and nappy rash cream within reach. Bath your baby every night and *never* shower your baby—you could easily drop a slippery baby or slip while holding him.

Test the water temperature with your elbow and make sure it is 38°C before you put your baby in the bath. Then undress him, but leave the nappy on for now, just in case! Wrap him in a towel and hold him under your arm so his head is supported by your hand over the bath. Use a face washer to gently rub around the fontanel area, the soft spot on the baby's head, to prevent any cradle cap. Cradle cap is just a collection of skin, layer upon layer. Then bring him back to the table and gently dry his hair in a circular motion.

Now you can undo your baby's towel and take off the nappy. Pick your baby up with your hand under his head. The best way to hold a baby in the bath is to gently lie the baby on your wrist with your arm around the baby and your fingers grasping the arm. Hold both legs and gently settle the baby into the bath bottom first, lowering him very slowly into the bath until the water is just at his neck.

You can let the baby's legs go and let him float and enjoy the beautiful, warm water. Put your hand on his stomach to make him feel more secure.

If he cries, it may be because the water is too cold or too hot, or part of his upper body is wet and now exposed to the air.

Talk to your baby while you bath him . . . he knows your voice, he finds comfort in you being with him, and when he is calm in the warm bath he will open his eyes and look around. Gently wash him, especially under his arms, under his chin and around his genitals and buttocks.

When you think he's had enough, pat him dry, making sure you get under his arms and between all the creases

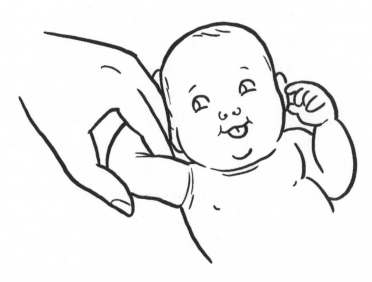

To dry under your baby's arm, lift the arm up by the elbow

(if you have two wet surfaces rubbing together, it can cause an infection). Lift his arm up by holding his elbow. If you try to lift his arm by the hand, he will instinctively pull it down.

When he is dry, put the nappy on first. This will prevent any mess and ensure you won't have to bath him again. Dress him and, finally, wrap him up using Cath's Wrap. Your baby is now ready for feeding.

Ears, eyes, noses, mouths, chins and bottoms

A little baby has lots of skin rolls, creases and bits and pieces. I was taught very early on in my midwifery education not to put anything smaller than your elbow in a baby's ear, nose, mouth or eye. These days professionals and pharmacists encourage parents to squirt saline up their baby's nose to remove mucus. If your baby has a stuffy or runny nose, you might be advised to suck out the mucus with a sucker, which amazes me. First of all, never do anything to your baby that you wouldn't do to yourself. If you're advised to squirt saline up your baby's nose, first squirt it up your own nose and see how uncomfortable it is, then use the sucker and you will see why the baby does not want you to use it—both are so uncomfortable. It will make your baby very unhappy, plus it is not necessary.

The hair in your baby's nose is both his body's defence against germs and provides additional humidity and moisture to inhaled air. Be patient. If your baby only has a runny nose, he's not sick. Just let him go, especially if he is your second, third or subsequent baby. A cold or a runny nose can be passed to him from the older children. On the other hand, first babies rarely get colds in the early weeks of life because parents are so protective of them. And that's nice.

As for baby's bottom, keep it clean and dry.

Circumcision is relatively uncommon these days, and is usually done for religious reasons. If your child is uncircumcised, you do not need to pull back his foreskin, which can cause trauma to the penis; instead, leave it alone and by the time the child is three or four years of age, he will probably play with his penis so much that the foreskin becomes naturally separated from the head of the penis. When your child is old enough, you can teach him general hygiene by pulling the foreskin back and cleaning underneath it while showering or bathing.

For girls, just clean the outside of the vulva; you don't need to clean inside the vulva or vagina. Sometimes girls have a mucousy, bloody discharge in the weeks following birth. This is normal and is a hormonal response to birth.

Twins

For comprehensive advice on coping with twins for the first six weeks, see *TFSW*, pages 181–93.

3

Your baby's health

The health of your baby is paramount and as parents you know your baby the best. If you feel your baby is unwell, see your GP and have him checked. Especially when he is a young baby—they may get sick quickly, but they get better quickly!

The maternal and child health nurse

When your baby was born, a paediatrician would have checked him thoroughly for any obvious physical abnormalities and asked you a number of questions—for example, were there any difficulties with the birth; are you breast- or bottle-feeding, or both (see *TFSW*, page 40). Your council/ MCH nurse should also have examined him at the first and subsequent visits.

The MCH nurse plays an important role in your baby's health for the early years of his life. This service is free in Australia, but access will vary from state to state. To find out about the MCH service in your area, contact your local council. Whether your baby was born in hospital or at home, the service will be notified of the birth.

The MCH nurse will contact you to make an appointment for the initial visit, either in your home or at the local centre, which is a great place to meet other new mums within your area. Your MCH nurse will help you maintain your baby's health book and provide you with information and support on such issues as breastfeeding, immunisation, safe sleeping, the development of your baby, and mothers' groups (see page 87).

Immunisation

The immunisation programs around Australia help immunise children from an early age to protect them from serious illnesses in childhood.

Timing

The immunisation program starts at birth, with the baby's first hepatitis B injection. A second round of immunisation happens at six weeks and one day, but exceptions may be made for premature, sick or immunosuppressed children. Always check with your doctor if you have any concerns.

The spacing between immunisations is really important, so if you start the immunisation later, the baby still needs the same interval between each immunisation. For catch-up immunisations, please check with your local council or GP. Serious side effects or allergic reactions to immunisation are rare.

Use paracetamol, given according to the baby's weight and age, if the baby is uncomfortable or grizzly post-immunisation.

Most immunisations are free in Australia and there are always new immunisations available, so check with your GP for up-to-date information. It is also important for adults to be up to date with their immunisations, including whooping cough, especially when a new baby is due. Immunisation immunity decreases with age and we need constant protection. If in doubt at all, check with your GP, as a blood test can assess your immunisation status.

By law, immunisations must be up to date before your child starts childcare and kindergarten, or enrols in primary school.

Childhood schedule of immunisation from birth to four years

The information given in the tables below is reproduced from the National Immunisation Program Schedule: https://beta.health. gov.au/topics/immunisation/immunisation-throughout-life/ national-immunisation-program-schedule

Birth

Disease	Vaccine	Comments
An injection for hepatitis B[a] (usually offered in hospital)	*H-B-Vax® II Paediatric* or *Engerix B—Paediatric*	Hepatitis B vaccine should be given to all infants as soon as practicable after birth. The greatest benefit is if it is given within 24 hours, and it must be given within 7 days.

Two months

These vaccines can be given from six weeks of age.

Disease	Vaccine	Comments
A combined injection for diphtheria, tetanus, whooping cough (pertussis), hepatitis B, polio, Hib (haemophilus influenzae type b)	*Infanrix® hexa*	None
An injection for pneumococcal	*Prevenar 13®*	None
Oral drops for rotavirus	*Rotarix®*	Oral dose of rotavirus vaccine at 6–14 weeks of age

4 months

Disease	Vaccine	Comments
A combined injection for diphtheria, tetanus, whooping cough (pertussis), hepatitis B, polio, Hib (haemophilus influenzae type b)	*Infanrix® hexa*	None
An injection for pneumococcal	*Prevenar 13®*	None
Oral drops for rotavirus	*Rotarix®*	Oral dose of rotavirus vaccine at 10–24 weeks of age

6 months

Disease	Vaccine	Comments
A combined injection for diphtheria, tetanus, whooping cough (pertussis), hepatitis B, polio, Hib (haemophilus influenzae type b)	*Infanrix® hexa*	None

Disease	Vaccine	Comments
An injection for pneumococcal	*Prevenar 13®*	Medically at-risk children only
		Refer to the current edition of the Australian Immunisation Handbook for all medical risk factor conditions.

12 months

Disease	Vaccine	Comments
A combined injection for measles, mumps, rubella	*M-M-R® II* or *Priorix®*	None
An injection for meningococcal ACWY	*Nimenrix®*	None
An injection for pneumococcal	*Prevenar 13®*	None

Before immunisation

Tell the doctor/nurse if your child:

- is unwell (has a temperature over 38.5°C)
- has had a severe reaction following any vaccine
- has had any severe allergic reactions to any other medication or substances
- has had any vaccine in the past month

- has had an injection of immunoglobulin or received any blood products or a whole blood transfusion within the past year
- was a preterm infant born at less than 32 weeks gestation, or weighed less than 2 kilograms at birth
- has had an intussusception (a blockage caused by one portion of the bowel sliding into the next piece of bowel, like the pieces of a telescope)
- has a chronic illness
- has a bleeding disorder
- does not have a functioning spleen
- lives with someone with a disease or who is having treatment that causes lower immunity
- is having treatment that causes low immunity (such as oral steroid medication, radiotherapy or chemotherapy)
- identifies as an Aboriginal or Torres Strait Islander.

Flat head syndrome

One of the guidelines on reducing the risk of SIDS encourages all parents to put their babies to sleep on their backs from birth. When doing this, a baby sleeps for a long time on his back and he may develop a flat spot on the back or the side of his head. This is called plagiocephaly, or flat head syndrome. From birth, the baby's skull bones are soft and mouldable, and if he is lying in the same position for long periods, the affected part of his head will flatten. This can happen within weeks after birth.

Pressure from lying on his back causes the head to look misshapen, with ears and forehead looking 'different'.

Babies can also be born with an odd-shaped head, often due to the position in which the baby was lying in utero.

Who can help

Talk to your MCH nurse, GP or paediatrician, who can assess the baby's head and, if necessary, refer you to a paediatric physio for assessment. As prevention is better than cure, I encourage tummy time for babies from day one.

Another issue that can cause concern is if the baby's head is turning consistently to one side. Again, this is often due to the baby's position in utero. You MCH nurse, GP or paediatrician will give you a referral to a paediatric physio who will teach you gentle massage techniques to resolve the tightness. It's also good to place the baby facing in different directions on the floor, or even in the cot. If he is lying on the floor and any stimulation—for example, a window—is on the right, the next time you're putting him down for back time or tummy time, lay him on the floor so he has to turn his head facing to the left. Tummy time, back time and massage all help.

Hip dysplasia of the newborn

Hip dysplasia (DDH) is more common in babies who have been in a breech position—that is, in an upright position—in utero. It is common in first-born children, girls more than boys and babies whose siblings or parents have a history of hip dysplasia. One or both hips can be affected.

During pregnancy, women have a high level of relaxin, a hormone in their blood to help their ligaments stretch during pregnancy and birth. It also helps the pelvis stretch during the birthing process to allow the baby through. Some of this hormone can also enter the baby's bloodstream, allowing the baby's hip joint to become loose in its socket.

Symptoms

- During the newborn check, the doctor or midwife/MCH nurse may feel a clunk or a click in one or both hips.
- The baby's legs are different lengths when stretched out straight.
- The baby may have uneven creases or fat folds at the backs of his legs.

Treatment

Most doctors order a scan of the baby's hips at six weeks of age if the baby is clinically at risk, in other words, if there was breech presentation during pregnancy, if there is a family history of hip dysplasia or if the paediatrician feels a 'click' or 'clunk' on examination. A hip brace may be recommended to keep the hips in the correct position and ensure the ligaments tighten around the hip joint. Other cases of DDH may need a hip spica plaster cast that covers both legs from the ankles to the abdomen.

Depending on the baby's condition, the brace may stay on for six weeks to six months. Usually the brace stays on for 24 hours a day but in some cases it can be removed for the daily bath. You can change your baby's nappies without removing the brace. A scan will be done initially and after the baby has worn the brace for the recommended period, the doctor orders an X-ray to check the hip is in the correct position before removing the brace. The good news is that in 2018 the success rate of braces is excellent.

Rashes

There are a number of skin rashes your baby might have in his first 12 months.

Erythema toxicum, a common rash affecting most full-term babies, is due to a maternal hormonal response after birth. It's usually a flat red patch with some little bumps and sometimes pustules. It usually starts on day 4 or 5, although it can appear as late as three to six weeks of age. It typically appears first on the face, then spreads to the upper trunk, the lower legs and arms. The palms and soles of the feet are not affected. Resist the urge to squeeze the pustules and only use water on the rash. It will disappear without treatment.

Neonatal milia are harmless small white cysts that cover the nose. Again, just wash the affected skin with water. They will disappear spontaneously after four to six weeks.

Pityrosprum folliculitis, commonly known as milk spots, are due to increased activity of the newborn's sebaceous glands, which causes inflammation. They look like pimples and usually appear on the nose and forehead, and often prominently on the cheeks. The rash will resolve itself so, again, don't squeeze the spots. Just wash with warm water.

For more on your baby's skin, see *TFSW*, pages 239–42.

Reflux

If your baby is uncomfortable, miserable and unhappy, and cries and cries and cries, it's more than likely he's suffering from the dreaded reflux, which is like constant heartburn in adults.

It's very distressing for new parents, who will often take advice from well-meaning friends and family who decree that the baby has 'colic' or 'bad wind'. A lot of money may then be spent on over-the-counter medicines. Unfortunately, the reflux will only get worse until it is treated properly by your GP or paediatrician, so please seek medical advice.

At the top of the stomach there is a sphincter that keeps food down when we swallow. The stomach also produces acid juices to help break down food so it can be digested. Some newborn babies have a floppy or immature sphincter and when some milk comes up, the acid in the stomach comes up too, causing heartburn.

When he's feeding, a baby with reflux struggles and fusses at the breast or bottle, arching his back and moving his head around, but you may think he's just refusing the breast. He will cry, and when he finally falls asleep and is put in his cot, he will start crying again within five minutes, inconsolable until fed again . . . and so the process goes on, and on.

Often babies suffering from reflux vomit. It's not a large amount of vomit, and it's not all the milk the baby has just had, but it will be enough to make you feel concerned. Although babies with reflux seem generally unhappy, they are actually well. Babies with reflux do not always lose weight; in fact, some actually gain a lot of weight, as feeding is a comfort for them.

Other common symptoms of reflux include your baby:

- being unable to lie on his back without crying
- drawing up his knees
- waking up from a deep sleep screaming
- burping and looking as if he has eaten something he doesn't like; it's actually the acid in his stomach refluxing up.

Reflux is very distressing for everyone. Your once calm and sleeping baby neither feeds well at the breast nor sleeps, and he cries most of the day. He also loves being held upright so you'll spend 20 hours a day on your feet, walking him. The symptoms of reflux can appear as early as week 2 or 3.

Treatment

First, it's important to have reflux diagnosed by a medical professional. Your doctor will prescribe medicine, which can take up to a week to work. Initially, often an antacid is used in conjunction with the medicine.

Only give your baby medicine that has been prescribed by your doctor after a physical check.

Teething

It's not hard to tell when your baby starts teething. He may be irritable during the day and sleepless at night. (And you might be too!) Here's what to expect and how to keep your baby comfortable.

Your baby was born with all 20 primary teeth below his gum line. They typically start to come through between six and 12 months, and you should expect your child to have his full set of baby teeth in place by the age of three.

What's normal when teething?
- red cheek or ear
- rubbing of ears
- waking at night
- irritability
- fussiness with food
- dribbling more than usual

What's abnormal when teething?

- fever
- vomiting
- diarrhoea
- rash all over the body

How to treat teething pain

Babies who are teething need lots of love and cuddles. You have to understand how much discomfort they are in. If your baby has problems taking paracetamol, an anti-inflammatory medicine is really helpful, as it not only decreases the pain but also helps soothe any inflammation. Make sure you follow the instructions on the package according to your baby's age and weight.

Teething rings are fabulous for easing your baby's pain and discomfort. Buy a few so you can keep at least one of them cold in the fridge while he uses the other one.

In my opinion, teething gels are not that helpful. It's best to give medicine, such as paracetamol.

Teething was very challenging for my two children, in particular my first child, who started teething quite young. It was a combination of very red cheeks and runny poo, but the tell-tale sign was how upset he was when teething. This seemed to start happening before there were any signs of teeth! However, the teeth always appeared soon after. It took me some time to recognise the distinct link between the pain he was experiencing and teething. It was definitely a challenging time for my first child. Teething seems to vary from one child to the next, with our second child teething much later. The pain was definitely still there for her too (just more spread out over time . . .).

— BRYDIE

Tongue-tie

About 5 per cent of babies have mild tongue-tie or ankyloglossia, which is a congenital, thick piece of skin connecting the tongue to the floor of the mouth under the tongue, resulting in its reduced mobility. It is now nearly routine practice for some paediatricians, midwives and lactation consultants to encourage new parents to let a trained professional snip the tie with a pair of sterile scissors and/or laser soon after birth.

Some professionals tell new parents that tongue-tie is to blame for sore nipples, their baby not sucking, and potential speech problems when the child is older. I have consulted with experienced obstetricians; ear, nose and throat surgeons; oral and maxillofacial surgeons; and dentists about this, and they all agree that it is a totally unnecessary and invasive procedure for newborn babies.

In severe cases, where the tongue is split at the tip, an oral and maxillofacial surgeon will recommend you wait until your child is older, when the lower anterior teeth have preferably erupted, before the tongue-tie is excised under a general anaesthetic.

So be patient. But if you have issues with your baby attaching, please use nipple shields first (see page 88 for more information). It adds length to the nipple and enables the baby to suck. Likewise, if your baby is bottle-fed, the long teat will enable him to feed successfully.

For expert advice on why you should delay snipping the tie, see *TFSW*, page 49.

Vitamin D drops

If your vitamin D levels have been low during pregnancy and you are breastfeeding, your baby will need to be given vitamin D drops. It's easy to apply vitamin D drops—simply place the drops on your baby's tongue. If you are bottle-feeding your baby, the formula has all the vitamin D required for a baby and you won't need to give him a supplement.

Wee and poo

Plenty of wet nappies mean your baby is well hydrated. If the nappies are dry or your baby has not passed urine, seek medical advice.

A fully breastfed baby will have runny, yellow poo, and they can poo before, during and after every feed, but some breastfed babies can go for more than 10 days without pooing at all. A breastfed baby is never constipated, so as long as the baby is feeding well and passing wind, the poo will follow.

If your baby's poo is black, red or white, you should consult your doctor. Black (not meconium, which the baby produces after birth) could mean he has some internal bleeding high in his gut. Red poo can indicate an allergy to cow's milk protein, or a bowel complication called intussusception (when the bowel telescopes in on itself, resulting in 'redcurrant jelly poo'). If his liver isn't producing enough bile, his poo will be white, and if the flow of bile is blocked and not draining from the liver, your baby's poo will be pale, grey or clay-coloured. In all these cases, take a photo of the soiled nappy, put it in a plastic bag and show it to your doctor.

Blood in the baby's poo

Cow's milk protein is one of the most common causes of food allergies in newborn babies. If you notice blood in the baby's poo, either take a photo of the blood-stained poo or put the nappy in a plastic bag and take it with you when you see the doctor. If you are breastfeeding, the paediatrician will encourage you to eliminate dairy from your diet. If your child is allergic to cow's milk, be careful to avoid milk and all milk-containing foods.

If the baby continues to have blood in his poo, your paediatrician will advise you to put him on a prescription formula and express your milk until his bowel actions settle down. I'm afraid the prescription formula smells foul (and so does the baby's poo) but he will drink it happily.

If your baby has any signs of gastroenteritis, your doctor may ask for a sample of the baby's poo to send to pathology for testing.

Wind

Burping and hiccuping are normal body processes. So is wind. It does not make your baby sick, nor is it extremely painful. Often feeding will help the baby with what we call 'the oral/ anal reflex'—that is, when the baby sucks either at the breast or on a bottle, the anus is stimulated and will expel what the body does not need anymore (poo), making room for more food (milk) to be ingested for growth.

Worms

I know it sounds revolting but kids can get worms, especially when they are mixing with other children or going to childcare. In Australia, threadworm (also known as pinworm) is the most common type of worm in children and adults. They won't hurt you or your child, and they're simple to treat, but they are also easily spread between humans.

Children get worms when they put their hands to their mouths and swallow an egg, which can be found in dust, toys and bed linen. Once swallowed, the egg gets into the small gut where the worms hatch and lay more eggs around the child's anus. I know it's gross, but we need to understand these issues. If your child often has an itchy bottom, especially at night-time, chances are he has worms. He will scratch his bottom and then inevitably put his hand to his mouth—and the cycle repeats. Worms can affect sleep, eating and behaviour, too, so its a good idea to worm children routinely—at least every six months. The good news is that the treatment is a chocolate-like square.

Tips for treating and preventing worms

- Speak to your pharmacist about the most common treatment for worms.
- Everyone in the family needs to be treated—both parents and children—but *not* newborn babies.
- At the same time, worm any animals in the household.
- Wash all the bed linen.
- It's vital to keep your children's nails trimmed at all times. I often recommend doing this in the bath, and then washing your children's hands with soap before soaking them in the water.

My 10-month-old child was waking up at night frequently. Midwife Cath told me to treat the whole family for worms with chocolate squares. I must say I had never heard of it before! I was advised to wash all the linen, cut my children's nails in the bath, wash their hands and nails with soap and water, and give them a good soaping up, all over, in the bath. I did all of those things (it was a big day), and then we repeated the cycle two weeks later. To my horror, when my child did a poo the next day I saw the worms in her poo!!!!! We now treat the whole family on a regular basis. Before, my child was waking up two to three times a night. Just treating the worms changed her sleep behaviour.

— VIOLET

When to seek medical advice

Look at your baby. He will show you what he's feeling. If he's turning his nose up and screwing up his face, it's just because he can! He is not sick. If your baby is sick, his body will declare it, and you will recognise the signs.

I've repeated the following section from *TFSW*, as it's so important to be aware of when you should be concerned about your baby.

Go to the doctor or a hospital if your baby:

- is floppy or unresponsive
- has jerky movements
- has watery diarrhoea
- is a blue or dusky colour
- has a high temperature, over 38.5°C
- is not feeding well
- is constantly vomiting, or projectile vomiting
- is not producing a lot of wet nappies
- has blood in his poo
- is crying uncontrollably and you cannot stop or settle him
- is coughing constantly.

You don't need to worry about your baby if he:

- is burping
- has wind or is farting
- has lots of wet nappies
- has pooey nappies
- brings up a small amount of vomit
- has the hiccups
- is alert
- is looking around and not crying.

4

Speech, language and communication

Thanks to speech pathologists Elise Swallow and Nichols Pakkiam for contributing this chapter.

Early communication development

Language development is a unique and beautiful experience that starts our lifelong desire to connect and share with others through interactions. This experience occurs as early as when the foetus's senses begin to develop by week 18 of pregnancy. From then on, noises become more audible and sensitive, which proceeds to familiarity with speech and language. By the time a baby is born, he will already be familiar with responding to noises and sounds.

Babies learn to communicate. Many skills are required in order to interact verbally but the three obvious ones are communication, language and speech. These three areas develop together but can be discussed separately, in order to help us understand what is going on.

Communication

Communication is an exchange of information. From birth, babies use their bodies to communicate. They won't come up with words until they're about 10 to 14 months of age. Before this they use crying, cooing, eye gazing, facial expressions, laughing and body movements to communicate their needs and feelings.

In the first six to eight months of life your baby's behaviour is not under his control; it is hardwired in. Communication is one behaviour they learn to control over this time; it develops through an adult interpreting their hardwired communication and responding to their needs. As a parent you can often feel as if you're always guessing what your child needs. It takes time to learn what your baby is trying to communicate through his behaviour. After a lot of trial and error, you can learn what your baby is saying through his cries, cooing, eye gaze, facial expressions, laughing and body movements. By *you* responding to these cues, your baby is learning how to ask for things, protest against others, comment on experiences and play! This is how they learn how to connect their ideas or feelings to their actions. This is the backbone of all intentional behaviours.

Around six to 12 months of age, babies become intentional with their communication. Initially, while language is developing in their brains, they use 'non-verbal communication', such as eye contact, facial expressions, reaching and pointing to communicate.

Language

Language is the meaning behind words and phrases. It develops alongside communication in the brain from birth. So speaking to your baby from birth is vital for his language development. First, babies learn what words mean—that is, comprehension—then they use words to speak—expression.

The lists that follow show how the development of comprehension and expression unfold during the first year of life.

Development of comprehension

BIRTH TO SIX MONTHS
- glances at a face momentarily when a person is talking to him
- shows enjoyment of attention by smiling
- reacts to sounds in the environment
- responds to, and turns towards, sounds
- puts objects in mouth

SIX TO 12 MONTHS

- begins understanding up to 50 words
- anticipates events and play
- shakes/bangs play items and toys
- looks for items/people that/who go out of sight
- starts responding to his name
- understands very simple instructions such as 'Come here'

Development of expression

BIRTH TO SIX MONTHS

- vocalises with varying pitch and volume
- smiles and cries
- starts babbling
- produces vegetative sounds such as coughs and sneezes
- coos and laughs
- produces repetitive babbling, such as 'mama', 'dada', 'tata'

SIX TO 12 MONTHS

- intent to request, refuse and comment emerges
- increases variety of vocalising and combination of babbling sounds
- attempts to imitate facial expressions
- seeks attention
- can handle back-and-forth communication
- tries to say some meaningful single words, although he doesn't get all the sounds right—for example, pronounces 'car' as 'tar'

Speech

Speech results from the movement of the speech muscles to produce sounds. These muscles are also used for eating and drinking. All movements in the body start off big and uncoordinated, then, as the nerves develop, the movements become precise and coordinated. Speech is one of the most complex series of movements the body performs, and it involves at least 100 muscles working together with speed and precision. Initially, movements of the head, neck and torso are controlled by reflexes (for example, suck-swallow-breathe when feeding) and eventually move to coordinated voluntary movements (for example, speaking). During the first year of life your child is exploring what his mouth can do while building strength and coordination so that he will eventually be able to speak, eat and drink easily. The precision of making sounds and words takes years to develop.

The following lists show how long the different pre-speech and speech movements take to develop. Some speech movements are easier than others, so their sounds develop earlier. Some movements are harder, thus their sounds take longer.

Hearing and understanding

BIRTH TO THREE MONTHS

- startles to loud sounds
- quiet smile when spoken to
- seems to recognise your voice

- increases or decreases sucking behaviour in response to sound

FOUR TO SIX MONTHS

- moves his eyes in the direction of sounds
- responds to changes in the tone of your voice
- notices toys that make a noise

SEVEN TO 12 MONTHS

- enjoys games like peekaboo
- turns and looks in the direction of sounds
- listens when spoken to
- recognises words for common items, such as 'cup', 'shoes', 'book' or 'milk'
- begins to respond to requests ('Come here please' or 'Would you like some more?')

Talking

BIRTH TO THREE MONTHS

- makes pleasure sounds (cooing, gooing)
- has different cries for different needs
- smiles when he sees you

FOUR TO SIX MONTHS

- babbling sounds more speech-like, with many different sounds, including 'p', 'b' and 'n'
- chuckles and laughs
- vocalises excitement and displeasure

- makes gurgling sounds when left alone and when playing with you

- babbling long and short groups of sounds, such as 'tata', 'upup' and 'bibibi'
- speech or non-crying sounds to get and keep attention
- uses gestures to communicate (waving, holding arms up to be picked up)
- imitates different speech sounds
- has one or two words—such as 'hi', 'dog', 'dada', 'mama'—around 12 months

Ways to help your baby learn to communicate

Face to face

Babies love faces and enjoy looking at them. A face provides a beautiful canvas for interaction, especially when it is rich with expression and care. Even though their vision is limited, babies are hardwired for social interaction from birth by being programmed to look at faces more than anything else. This is because our faces carry *huge* amounts of information that we may or may not realise we are expressing to others. Babies start recognising different faces from birth, as they learn who their caregivers are. They also start to learn what different facial expressions mean, and then start responding to them and copying them. This is a very important part of communication. You may enjoy watching your baby's responses when you make different facial expressions.

Babies also learn to speak by copying sounds they see and hear around them. For your baby to learn all this information, it is important for you to be in close face-to-face proximity to your baby when speaking to him. Whether you're holding your baby or not, about 20 centimetres is a good distance. You can tell if your baby can see you, as he will look straight at you and respond to what you are doing. Using a pram that's designed to have your baby facing towards you is a great way to facilitate more of this face-to-face time.

Baby talk

Also known as Motherese, baby talk is the high-pitched, lyrical 'baby talk' adults use when speaking to babies. It has been shown to improve language development in babies because the baby's brain is heightened to learn and retain information when adults speak in this style. Baby talk uses lots of interesting facial expressions, so it will also hold your baby's attention longer. Throughout their lives you will see that the more you can hold his attention, the more he will learn. To help his language development, we recommend using real words and phrases rather than made-up words with baby talk. You do not have to speak in this way all the time, just when it feels natural.

It is appropriate to use baby talk until your baby is about 10 to 12 months of age. Remember it is *baby* talk, not toddler talk.

Baby sign

Baby sign involves using a gesture instead of speech to communicate a word. Teaching your baby a gesture when saying a word helps him to understand what the word means. As simple hand control develops before speech control, he will sometimes use the gesture before being able to say the word. We don't recommend slaving away, trying to teach your baby lots of signs; just try a few to help his communication in the early stages. During the period between your baby understanding a word and being able to say it yet, these gestures can be very helpful stepping stones towards your baby not crying in frustration. You do not have to use specific sign language, just gestures that make sense to you and your baby. Make sure you tell other caregivers what they are too, so they can understand your baby's communication attempts. I would recommend teaching the following:

- 'up'—index finger points up
- 'want'—hand held out with palm facing up
- 'drink'—hand moves to the mouth as if holding a cup
- 'eat'—fingers move to lips as if holding sultanas
- 'stop'—hand pushes out to make a 'stop' sign
- 'finished'—rotating both hands clenched in fists.

You can model these signs for your baby from birth, but he won't pay much attention to them until he is around six months old. To teach your child, just use the sign at the exact time you say the word. For example:

Baby wants to be picked up
- stressing the 'up' and pointing fingers up when saying 'up', adult asks, 'You want to come **up**?'
- adults picks up child and says, 'Up!'

After modelling the sign and word to your child for a few months, you can gently show him how to do it. For example:

Baby wants to be picked up
- Stressing the 'up' and pointing fingers up when saying 'up', the adult asks, 'You want to come **up**?'
- Then the adult gently holds up the baby's arms, and says, 'Up!'

Adult gives the child three opportunities to use the gesture on their own:

- 'You want to come **up**?' Adult pauses.
- 'You want to come **up**?' Adult pauses.
- 'You want to come **up**?' Adult pauses.
- Adults picks up the child and says, 'Yes, up!'

Narrating

You can help your baby start to learn the meaning behind words for feelings, objects, people and experiences by narrating what he is interested in during the day. Being face to face is the richest way to do this, but even when you can't be right next to him, it is still helpful to talk about what is going on around him. Your baby has to learn the meaning of words in a meaningful context, long before he can say them. Even if you aren't exactly sure what he wants, just guess and say it anyway, as he loves to be spoken to. The key is to work out what he's interested in and say what you think he is trying to communicate.

Here are some simple examples of helping your baby learn the meaning behind words for certain feelings:

- Baby is grizzling when he is tired. Adult says, 'Oh, you're feeling tired. Let's get ready for a sleep.'
- Baby is crying because he is hungry. Adult says, 'I hear you crying. I think you're feeling hungry. Let's have some milk.'
- Baby is laughing because he is being tickled. Adult says, 'Oh, is that funny? You're feeling happy!'
- Baby is grizzling because he wants attention. Adult says, 'You're feeling bored. Do you want Daddy to play with you?'
- Baby is crying because a stranger has picked him up. Adult says, 'Are you feeling angry? You want your mummy.'

Below are two examples of learning the words for objects and people:

- Baby is playing with a rattle. Adult says, 'You're holding the rattle.'
- Baby is looking at his mother's face. Adult (mother) says, 'You're looking at Mummy!'

Here are two examples of learning the words for different experiences:

- Adult is changing the baby's nappy. Adult (father) says, 'You've done poos. I'm wiping your bottom. All nice and clean. Daddy is putting on a clean nappy.'
- Baby is being taken for a walk in the pram. Adult watches the baby's eye gaze and comments on what he is looking at. Adult says, 'We're walking with the pram. You're looking at the trees. A car just went by. Hello, lady.'

Babbling

Listening to baby sounds is one of the cutest and funniest experiences, and it represents an important milestone in your baby's life. Babbling is one of the first ways your baby learns to use his voice. Throughout his first year of life, babbling begins with uncoordinated, random sounds and proceeds to a variety of early sounds and repetition of sounds. Babbling is how your baby explores and strengthens his speech system. Alongside the intentional communication that we discussed, babbling becomes more consistent and precise from six to 12 months of age.

Tips for helping babbling

Promoting babbling is a great way to encourage shared communication and interaction. When you copy your baby's babbles, he gets a strong sense of empowerment and will want to speak more. He is also learning attention, imitation and turn taking. All these are important social skills.

You can promote interactions with your baby during babbling by simply repeating and imitating his babbling sounds. For example:

- Baby says 'awa' or 'ma ma ma ma'.
- Adult looks at the baby with a smile and says 'awa' or 'ma ma ma ma'.

Here are some other tips for helping your baby babble.

- Mimic your child's babbling during daily face-to-face routines, such as mealtimes, nappy changes or when having a cuddle.
- Asking your baby simple questions and commenting on what's happening are great ways to get his attention and provide babbling opportunities.

- When he babbles, pause before copying him. Pausing shortly between turns provides a great space and opportunity for engagement or continuing an interaction.
- Once your baby has babbled the same sounds for a while, vary the sounds you babble so he can learn new sounds.

The 'one-up rule'

This rule involves adding in the word your child needs to learn next. This helps your baby to say the actual words, not just know their meaning, as when narrating to them or copying your baby's sounds while babbling. You *only* use this once he starts using words in context. It is done in the same way as promoting babbling, except you use words instead. Once you hear your baby using single words in context, you can teach him new words by naming the things he is interested in.

For example:

- Baby sees a dog.
- Adult says, 'Dog.'

Once your child is easily using this word, copy him but add two words. For example:

- When the baby sees the dog, he quickly and effortlessly says, 'Dog.'
- Adult says, 'Yes, black dog.'

Once he is easily using two words, copy him but add three words. For example:

- When the baby sees the dog, he quickly and effortlessly says, 'Black dog.'
- Adult says, 'Yes, big black dog.'

You can keep doing this for the rest of your child's life to help him expand his vocabulary but, after a few years, if not before, I think he will be quite sick of you repeating what he says.

5

Looking after yourself

You don't realise how much work a baby is until you've had one, and then the constant feeding and sleep deprivation can come as a shock.

Give yourself a break

Days and nights can be long and isolating with a new baby, especially when your partner goes back to work. A few basics will really help:

- Have a shower and get dressed first thing every morning.
- Eat breakfast every morning and keep your fluids up.
- Limit visitors in the early days and weeks—learn to say a guilt-free 'no'.
- As you and your baby start to get some sleep, take a walk each day.

- Arrange to have coffee or lunch with a friend.
- Arrange for a relative to mind the baby while you have your hair done.
- Have a rest when your baby does.
- Have a date night with your partner every now and then. Ask someone you trust to look after the baby and go out for a quick meal or a movie. It's amazing how much better you'll feel after a break from the constant routine.

Family helpers

When your baby was first born you may have felt overwhelmed by eager grandparents and other loved ones who wanted to help with the baby and various domestic chores. If you've grown up in a big family you might love all the company and attention, but for others it can become quite stressful having people around all the time, especially as you are still getting to know your baby and perhaps adjust to being a parent for the first time.

Grandparents can provide unconditional love and play a key role in your child's life, and may eventually look after your baby or toddler when you go back to work. Of course, much depends on your own relationship with your parents and parents-in-law. If you're uncomfortable with the level of help on offer—either too much or too little—consider talking to them about it, or even writing down the things you really need help with.

When my first child was born, his paternal grandparents had retired to another state. It had been more than 10 years since their last grandchild was born and my mother-in-law was desperate to have a major role in looking after her six-week-old grandson, even on short visits. She would swoop on him for a cuddle as soon as he woke up, but after a few minutes he'd start to cry because he was hungry. It was stressful, but I didn't think I could say anything when she saw him so infrequently.

One afternoon David was crying in her arms in the next room and I heard my father-in-law say to her, 'I think you should give him to his mother.' I was gobsmacked to hear her reply, 'What can she do for him that I can't?' I knew that, years before, she had spent night after night soothing her first grandchild, who screamed all night with 'colic', so his mother could get some sleep, and I let it go. But I did rescue my baby after a few minutes!

— ANN

It's also good to bear in mind that parenting styles change over the generations, so you may need to explain the Red Nose guidelines in relation to your baby's sleep position, for example, or point out that it's no longer advised to put your bare-legged baby in his pram down at the bottom of the garden so he can 'play in the sun'. Also, ask your parents and parents-in-law to be immunised against whooping cough and, if they smoke, let them know that you don't allow smoking in your home or around your baby.

Australia is a multicultural country, and many people traditionally practise cultural confinement—for 40 days the new mother and her baby stay at home where they are cared for by other women in the extended family. For more information, see *TFSW*, page 229.

Mothers' groups

Mothers' groups are held within the community and are often organised by the local MCH nurse or equivalent in your state. The group is open to first-time mothers and their babies, and is geared to educating new parents on the parenting issues they will face in the first 12 months—such as feeding the baby, safety, sleep and settling, and community events. Mothers' group is the time to make friends with other mothers within your local area; they often become friends for life. In many cases, children who start in mothers' groups together often end up going to the same kinder or the same school and become lifelong friends.

If you feel you are not ready to join a mothers' group, if your baby is really unsettled and you don't feel confident enough to attend, wait until he is older—perhaps three months—and then join. I find it's better to attend with an older, more settled child than with a two- to three-week-old crying baby. You will feel more confident taking your little one into a group of new mums as, by that time, you will know your baby, you are through those sleepless early nights and you are ready to participate and enjoy the group.

Breast care

Every mother and her baby are individuals, and I make sure that what I do is working for that particular mother and her baby. Some women have an abundance of milk, which makes it easier for the baby to feed well, gain weight and sleep; others have less milk, or the milk comes in slowly and the babies need extra kilojoules besides breast milk.

Nipple shields

If you have short, flat or inverted nipples, your baby may not be able to latch on to your breast properly. But there is help available if you can't attach your baby to the breast, or if you have grazed, cracked and sore nipples. Nipple shields are a fabulous solution to this problem. These soft silicon shields fit over the nipple, providing protection for a sore nipple as well as adding length to short, flat or inverted nipples. They also allow breast milk to pool around cracked nipples and heal them quickly.

Usually by the time the baby is three months old or so, he has drawn out the nipple through constant sucking and is able to latch on to the mother's nipple directly.

So nipple shields can make the difference between breastfeeding and not breastfeeding.

Unfortunately, some midwives and lactation consultants discourage the use of nipple shields, but the alternative is to express the breast milk and give it to the baby in a bottle, or even a cup. This causes the new mother a lot of unnecessary anxiety.

Shooting nipple pain

Some women experience severe pain while breastfeeding, a needle-like pain that shoots up the nipple through the breast. It can even continue between feeds. Naturally, it can make even the thought of breastfeeding a very stressful prospect.

For some women, expressing helps reduce the pain, allowing the baby to still drink breast milk, but it is unsustainable. If you have nipple pain, try this simple method each time you experience it. It will at least reduce the severity of the pain and, in some cases, even make it go away.

- Place your open hand over your breast with your nipple in the centre of your hand.

- Then gently but firmly press your breast into your back so you flatten the breast for 50 to 60 seconds. The pain will decrease and may even go altogether.

In some cases, the pain may be caused by thrush. This can be treated by using oral antifungal tablets, which you can buy over the counter at a pharmacy. The tablets come one in a packet. Taking one tablet every second day for three days will help remove the pain of thrush. No creams need to be applied to the nipples.

Mastitis

Mastitis is an infection in the breast that can occur during breastfeeding. It usually spreads from a crack in the nipple but it can also be caused by taking the baby on and off the breast too many times during feeding, rather than letting the baby take the nipple into the back of his mouth. It doesn't happen to everybody, but for some women, unfortunately, it happens frequently, especially if their breasts are engorged with milk, or they massage or rub their breasts. Women with mastitis feel terribly ill and can become sick very quickly.

It is important to know the signs of mastitis so you can catch it early. Often the first signs are a headache and a sore throat, along with a red, hot area on the breast that causes the mastitis. You can also experience flu-like symptoms such as hot and cold flushes, aches and joint pain, shivers, shakes and a feeling of general malaise. This feeling can take over within minutes and you feel very sick, very quickly. As soon as you see a red mark on your breast, see your doctor. Try not to wait until you feel very sick.

You will need pain-relief tablets and anti-inflammatory tablets as well as antibiotics—all prescribed by your doctor. Never take anyone else's medication.

It's very hard when you have mastitis, because you still need to feed your baby. Even though you feel unwell and your breasts are sore, you need to keep breastfeeding because the milk needs to continue to flow. It's very important to have the baby suck on the nipple that has mastitis, to ensure the milk is always 'moving'. Don't feed one side only as the brain does not discriminate when it lets the milk down, filling both breasts ready for the baby to suck.

Do not massage your breasts or put hot packs on them when you have mastitis. This is a common practice encouraged by some practitioners but, in my experience, massaging the breast actually makes things worse. Instead, put on a firm bra without an underwire, take your medication and let the baby feed. Clean, cold (stored in the freezer) cabbage leaves flowered around your breast will provide tremendous relief. You may need to remove any large veins from the leaves so they sit well on your breasts.

Once you start antibiotic and anti-inflammatory therapy prescribed by your doctor, you should start to feel better within 24 hours. If you don't feel any change, go to your doctor or local hospital straight away, as an abscess can form, making you extremely ill. Trust your body. If you don't feel well, tell somebody and get help.

Wrist pain when feeding

Some women experience tremendous pain in their wrists—not only carpal tunnel syndrome during pregnancy, but also de Quervain's syndrome of the wrist after the birth. The latter is a painful inflammation of the wrist that is often caused by repetitive movement, and nothing equals the repetitive movement of holding, feeding, handling and carrying a baby. De Quervain's syndrome is caused by the tendons at the base of the thumb becoming inflamed, putting pressure on the nerves and causing pain. The best thing to do is rest your wrist which, when you have a baby, is usually impossible, so a splint on the wrist can actually help immobilise the wrist and decrease the pain. If it continues, you can consult a hand surgeon. You may need to have an injection of a painkiller, such as cortisone, into the wrist.

Abdominal muscles after birth

Surprisingly, about two thirds of mothers have some degree of abdominal muscle separation resulting from pregnancy. This can be seen both during pregnancy as a dome or ridge in the upper abdomen, and following delivery, as a sense of looseness, or widening. This is often unavoidable due to the abdominal muscles needing to accommodate the growing baby, however, there are ways to prevent the separation worsening. As the stomach muscles stretch, the connective tissue that joins them in the middle may separate a little, right where the two sides of the 'six pack' muscles join together. This separation can cause what looks like a small gutter in the middle of the abdomen when bending forwards, and is commonly known as a diastasis recti (DRAM). Factors that may contribute to DRAM include hormonal changes and abdominal wall weakness.

Prevention of DRAM

Together with pelvic floor exercises, specific core strengthening exercises prescribed by a physiotherapist can be helpful in preventing DRAM. Pilates and yoga can also be very helpful in strengthening the deep abdominal muscles, while teaching awareness of posture and appropriate movements.

Exercises to avoid

Avoid anything that increases the pressure in your abdomen, such as straining on the toilet or heavy coughing, without first activating your pelvic floor to support the downward pressure. Any exercise that flexes the spine or flexes the six pack muscles, such as sit-ups or crunches, should be avoided unless specifically prescribed by a health practitioner. Many boot camp or High Intensity Interval Training classes that promote weight loss and 'getting fit', unless instructed by a trained professional, can actually make abdominal separation worse and may lead to other complications over time.

Having sex again

You will have sex again!

It is recommended you wait until you have stopped bleeding and had your six-week postnatal check with your obstetrician before you resume sexual relations with your partner. Don't be surprised if for weeks after the birth you're convinced that this will never happen again! Often you feel anxious and vulnerable (and with good reason) after giving birth—not only vaginally, but after a C-section too. You are also so tired and sex is last on your list of things to do! You fall into bed, pyjamas on, and you wake up when the baby wakes you up! When they finally think about sex, some women get a bit worried and avoid it.

When I was a young midwife, an older obstetrician told me the vagina is a very 'forgiving area'. Give yourself time to heal and rest, and when the right time comes, make sure you use plenty of lubricant and try to relax and enjoy!

The physical effect of breastfeeding hormones causes the vagina to feel dry and in turn can make sex painful. Plus, when breastfeeding you can leak breast milk while having sex. I know it all sounds really romantic doesn't it! Take your time, there is no hurry and you are not going to do any damage to your vagina. If you find it's too painful, though, see your obstetrician and ask if there are any structural problems resulting from a vaginal delivery.

My top tips for resuming sex are the following:

- have the baby well fed and asleep
- relax
- take things slowly
- have a bottle of lubricant handy so things just glide
- try different positions.

Feeling angry with your baby

Due to sleep deprivation and various difficulties after the birth of their child, or even resulting from a difficult birth, some women can feel angry with their baby—especially if he is crying all the time, not sleeping and not feeding well. For new mums it can be a really difficult, isolating and confusing time. So many people tell us it's a great experience, and that we will always love our baby, and so much on social media points to skinny, happy mums with smiling, well-dressed, well-fed and sleeping babies. In the early weeks of becoming a parent, most women will at some point feel they cannot cope. It is best to get psychological help when the baby is little and your parenting is in the early stages as the issues just continue mount.

If you feel angry with your baby, the best thing to do is put him safely into his cot, walk away, take a few deep breaths and perhaps call a friend or your partner and explain how you are feeling. Remember, the baby isn't trying to make you feel unhappy or angry; he doesn't have the developmental understanding to make you feel upset. But the combination of his consistent crying and your sleep deprivation can really push your buttons and your limits to the edge. Always reach out for help: there are plenty of professionals online, as well as phone services and local hospitals (see 'Seeking help', page 239). Rather than hide how you're feeling, because you're embarrassed or ashamed, just tell someone how you feel and get some help.

Anxiety in parenting

We write and talk a lot about the physical side of parenting, but often don't pay enough attention to the psychological side. It's hard to prevent anxiety in parenting—especially in those early weeks when your hormones are out of control and you're extremely sleep deprived—but it's important to at least discuss the triggers that affect our early days as parents. I think in pregnancy and early parenting we are so vulnerable as women; we are often emotional when we are growing a baby, and then after the birth, when we begin parenting and are faced with trying to keep our baby safe, we can at times feel so irrational.

Often, it's best to do your own thing and work out what suits you and your baby. Respond to your baby the way you feel you should. If you have too many people in your head giving you advice, you will never find your own way through this fog of information. But remember, there is always help around—for example, mothers' groups and playgroups run by your local council can provide wonderful support (see page 87).

Look around for a professional with whom you have a comfortable rapport. If you have experienced clinical anxiety and/or depression prior to pregnancy, ensure you discuss this with your GP, obstetrician or midwife so you can arrange care during your pregnancy. It's also important to have some follow-up care in the early weeks after the baby has been born. You may need to stay on medication during pregnancy and your child's early years, but you must be under the care of a medical professional.

People with generalised anxiety disorder in parenting experience excessive anxiety and worry, often a lot about their own health. This worrying goes on every day, possibly all day.

It disrupts social activities and interferes with parenting and family. Adults with anxiety experience the following symptoms:

- restlessness
- constant tiredness
- difficulty concentrating, or mind going blank
- irritability
- difficulty sleeping—head racing, cannot sleep, sleeping short times only, although really tired.

For expert advice on anxiety and postnatal depression, see *TFSW*, pages 210–17.

PART 2
AFTER SIX WEEKS

There isn't anything quite like early parenting. The love you have for your child, the respect you have for each other as parents, and then doing all of this while sleep deprived—well, it's amazing! While you are in the eye of the storm you feel like you will never live a normal life or sleep again—I'm here to tell you you will, it gets easier, it gets better, the baby grows and the baby sleeps. Then you have another baby!

6

Seven to eight weeks

I'm almost eight weeks old. Daddy is so good at bathing me—he sings funny songs, too. Tummy time makes me hungry and then I sleep well for you. I love our cuddles—especially just the two of us at night. I love you Mummy.

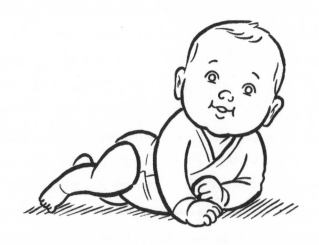

My book *The First Six Weeks* (*TFSW*) is an essential companion to this chapter, as it provides a detailed guide that will help you navigate the important first six weeks of your child's life.

In this chapter, I'll highlight some of the key points and best practices that are provided in detail in *TFSW* and, where appropriate, let you know where you can find more detailed information in that book. I'll also provide some new information to round off what you need to know to get you through these first eight weeks.

Feeding your baby

In the first eight weeks, milk—that is, breast milk and/or formula—is the only food you give your baby.

To have a healthy, happy baby, you need to feed him, and feed him constantly. How much babies need to feed in these early weeks can be a shock to new parents. If you think about it, from day 1 you have a newborn baby at about 3.5 kilograms, and within 12 months you have a toddler of 12 to 15 kilograms—cruising, or even running, around the room. The only way the baby is going to become a healthy, vigorous toddler is by drinking milk, and a lot of it.

Whether a baby is born little or big, he will be hungry. You cannot overfeed a baby but you *can* underfeed a baby. As I mentioned in Chapter 2, some underfed babies are diagnosed with colic, reflux and allergies, and professionals tell the mothers the babies have 'an incorrect latch'. They are *so* hungry. Make sure you feed your baby enough!

When you're in hospital for those first three to four days, you receive advice from well-trained midwives whose intentions are good. The only problem is that their advice is correct for those few days only. Your baby is going to grow, so their advice is not applicable as the baby grows, wakes up, and changes his feeding and sleeping patterns. And believe me, a six-, seven- or eight-week-old baby is very different to a baby who is one, two or three weeks old. The aim is long-term breastfeeding, and we must get it right in the early weeks so you have the confidence to continue feeding.

Understandably, new parents refer to what they learnt during those early days in hospital, and that becomes the model for how they care for their baby when they get home. I see this over and over again with my clients.

The danger of underfeeding a baby

I had a private consultation with a new mum whose five-day-old baby was born at about 2.8 kilograms. It was during a Melbourne summer and the little baby was dressed only in a singlet and nappy—no socks, top or wrap. You need to be careful not to underdress babies, especially when they had a low birth weight, like this one. This generation of mums are very aware of the SIDS guidelines and careful not to overheat babies, but I now often see babies that are underdressed. To overheat a baby you would need to fully dress him, and then put three or four blankets on top of him. I always like a newborn to be dressed in a singlet, nappy, onesie and a wrap—and that's for all seasons.

The mother was concerned about his crying, but he had not produced a heavy wet nappy since day 1. My extensive experience allows me to look at a baby and understand whether he is in proportion—that is, is he being fed well enough? This little baby was very long and very skinny. I suggested to the mother that she feed her baby while I sat with her. She looked at me and said, 'Okay, but he had a feed a couple of hours ago.' He hadn't been attaching correctly to the nipple, which meant he was not sucking well and therefore was not getting any fluids at all. The mum didn't have any fullness in her breasts and hadn't felt any fullness since she had given birth.

I was very concerned because I could see he was under-weight and underdressed, but explaining my concerns to a new mum is always really difficult. In my experience, babies of tall parents can be hungrier than usual. So I said to her, 'You know, if there are tall people in your family, your baby might need to be fed more frequently.' It turned out this baby did indeed have tall relatives on both sides of the family.

The mother was also very worried about her baby's lethargy and because he was only weeing urates, crystals that form from a combination of calcium and urate in urine. These crystals leave a red–orange stain in a baby's nappy. Any baby can pass urates, although he's more likely to do so when he is dehydrated because the urine becomes more concentrated. Weeing urates is most common when a baby hasn't been drinking enough breast milk and/or formula in the first few days of life. It's an indication that he needs something to drink.

This baby had also lost about 13 per cent of his birth weight. So the plan was to feed him formula for the next 24 hours and for the mother to express her milk to keep her supply up. Within 24 hours, and after two- to three-hourly formula feeds, the baby had produced one good wet nappy. He took 40 to 50 ml of formula every two hours. It took about two weeks for this baby to pass urine properly and gain an adequate amount of weight. After trying very hard, the mum didn't lactate and so she continued to bottle feed the baby. He is well and will continue to be well, but for his mum and dad it was a difficult introduction to parenthood.

So in these first eight weeks you need to feed the baby—a lot. If your baby is going from one breast to the other and back again in hospital and once you are home, and you feel as if you're getting nowhere, this is the time to give him formula. Not everyone has the same amount of milk in her breasts and it can sometimes take weeks for lactation to be established.

In the early days you just don't have 50 ml of milk in your breast to satisfy your hungry baby, especially boys!

As I say in *TFSW*, a baby needs food, love and warmth. I like to wrap babies for all feeds and all sleep, especially in the first six to eight weeks (see 'Cath's Wrap' on page 34). After that time, I tend to recommend feeding your baby without wrapping him, except for the last feed before you put him to sleep, whether it's during the day or at night-time.

Breastfeeding

Breastfeeding takes at least six weeks to establish and for the mother–baby connection to develop. So by the time your baby is seven or eight weeks old, things should be going smoothly. It is convenient, cheap and wonderful for both mother and baby, and once established is really very easy.

However, if you do not have enough milk, there really isn't much you can do. There is no tablet, food, biscuit, medicinal concoction or herb that will increase your supply. But try to persevere with breastfeeding and top up your baby with formula. Don't pump or express while also breastfeeding, as it will just take the milk from your breasts without making more. Expressing when you have a low supply can result in obsessive pumping that is neither physically nor emotionally sustainable. Expressing breast milk with a pump is only required if you have a sick or premature baby (see box, 'Expressing breast milk' over the page).

For further, comprehensive advice on successful breast-feeding, please see *TFSW*, pages 65–76 as well as pages 25–9 in this book.

Expressing breast milk

Expressing breast milk is the only way to maintain lactation when you and your baby are separated by illness, or when your baby has low weight or was born premature.

Even so, a breast pump is often on the top of new parents' 'to buy' list and, if you walk around a maternity ward, you will see a breast pump outside every room. New mums are being put on pumps as early as day 1—it's just not necessary. One mum told me she had a lovely vaginal birth and was giving her baby a breastfeed in the labour ward shortly after the birth. To her surprise one of the midwives went to hand express her other breast while she was breast feeding. I find this unbelievable. We need to be patient with a woman's body after she has a baby. It takes time for a new mother to lactate and learn how to breastfeed. Midwives should sit with the mother and her baby, teaching her the skills she needs to help the baby attach to the breast. The mother and baby need time to be together without the interference of a pump.

Of course you can breastfeed your baby without expressing once. None of the women I care for express or pump, and they go on to breastfeed long-term. Expressing milk every day simply causes anxiety. Midwives tell mothers to achieve a volume of milk they *must* express or pump frequently, so they sit on a breast pump instead of holding and loving their growing baby. Let your lactating brain do what Mother Nature intended and enjoy your baby. Be patient.

If a mother with a well baby expresses, the volume of milk she expresses will decrease over time. She will assume she doesn't have enough milk and will be more likely to give up breastfeeding.

Formula

I have provided detailed instructions on preparing formula on pages 32–3.

Breast milk or formula?

I've worked with mothers and babies for over 40 years, supporting every woman who wants to breastfeed, so I know that no two women lactate the same way. Unfortunately, the information given to women before the birth makes them think breastfeeding is easy. It isn't! To breastfeed successfully you need a lot of support, education and patience. There are times when women want to give up and stop—but with the correct support, encouragement and care, the hurdles that seem huge to the new mum can be overcome. When a mother is tired, sore, sleep-deprived and doesn't feel she is succeeding with breastfeeding, it is her support system of family and friends—or the voice in her head—that tells her to give up.

On the other hand, don't feel guilty if you can't—or simply don't want to—breastfeed your baby.

We know the majority of mothers intend to breastfeed, but if women experience problems and don't have ongoing support, especially from their partners, they will give up and formula-feed their baby. Our new mothers are receiving advice from hospital and from within the community that is leading to a sudden drop in breastfeeding once they are back at home with their new baby.

I know that not all women can or want to exclusively breastfeed, and I also know that introducing a bottle of formula early doesn't interfere with breastfeeding, in fact my patients breastfeed for longer—that is, up to and over twelve months. I'm sure it is because the partner does the BBB routine, offering one bottle of formula a night.

Women who have previously had breast surgery—for example, breast reduction or implants—do not lactate as well. Their milk will come in and they can feed initially, only to find they don't have enough breast milk for the growing baby.

I advise women who have had breast surgery not to expect to exclusively breastfeed. In my experience they definitely need to top the baby up with formula after most breastfeeds, especially for the first six to ten weeks. Initially they will be able to satisfy the baby with their breast milk but as the baby grows, they will need some formula to satisfy the baby's increased caloric needs. Doing so means they will breastfeed for longer too, as they will not have a hungry baby.

The mums I look after use one bottle of formula after the BBB routine at night, which does not affect their lactation, and I can confidently say they tend to breastfeed for longer, which is a fabulous win/win for both mother and baby. For the run-down on my bath, bottle and bed (BBB) routine, see pages 35–43.

Breast is best, and what is so fantastic about this slogan is that the community now understands that breast is indeed best. It doesn't mean, however, that the breast is the only way to give milk to a newborn baby.

Fed is best is perfect. It sends a supportive message to women who cannot or do not want to breastfeed and allows them to enjoy the wonderful early days and weeks of parenting while feeding their baby breast milk or formula, or a combination of both. But if you don't give your baby a bottle early enough in life, he will refuse it, and if you don't have enough milk this can lead to quite a few issues, including feeding aversion (see page 152). You will also have a big problem on your hands if you go back to work before he's weaned.

As long as the mother is happy and well, everyone is well.

The hungry baby

A hungry baby is awake, crying, searching with his mouth open from side to side, looking for a nipple to suck. He is well, but he is hungry. A baby who is hungry needs either breast milk or, if he has sucked long enough at the breast, a formula top-up. Feed him. You will see the difference once he has had a drink—he will sleep.

Don't replace milk with a dummy, as it does not have any kilojoules. As the baby sucks vigorously on the dummy it may settle him and stop him crying for a while, but it will not give him any food to help him grow, settle and be a happy baby who thrives and eventually sleeps well. A dummy should only be used to settle the baby to sleep once he has had enough to drink.

The baby's weight

A baby who is over a week old and feeding well should put on 100 to 150 grams per week. Some will gain less per week while others will put on much more. As long as the weight gain is consistent and the baby follows his percentile growth, there's nothing to worry about.

Don't be surprised if your baby's weight gain is not the same every week during weigh-ins with your maternal and child health nurse. Depending on his age and activity, each baby puts on different amounts weekly. Your baby cannot put on too much weight while breastfeeding or on formula milk. If your bottle-fed or breastfed baby has lots of fat rolls, don't worry—once he starts running around he will burn off his fat stores.

However, if your baby is consistently losing weight, seek professional advice.

Development

The percentile growth chart (see pages 232–37) in your baby's health book compares your child's weight, height and head circumference to other children of the same age and sex. This information enables your doctor or MCH nurse to assess how your baby is developing physically.

When comparing 100 babies of the same age on the percentile charts, if a baby is on the tenth percentile for weight, it means that 90 per cent of other babies at the same age weigh more and are longer than they are. A baby on the sixtieth percentile for height and weight is taller and heavier than 60 per cent of other babies.

Developmental milestones

Developmental milestones are behaviours or physical skills seen in babies, infants and children as they grow and develop. Every child develops at a different rate, so it's important not to compare your child to another child, even a sibling! Rolling over, crawling, walking and talking are all considered milestones. Babies at birth are capable of primitive movements and reflexes and, as they grow older, they learn different skills to survive. By 12 months of age the helpless newborn will be close to or even walking and saying a few words. The milestones are different for each age range.

There is a normal range in which a child may reach each milestone. For example, walking may begin as early as eight months in some children. Others walk as late as 18 months, which is still considered normal.

In the early years one of the reasons you visit the MCH nurse, or the equivalent in your state, is to monitor your child's growth and development. Most parents also look out for different milestones. If you have concerns about your child's development, talk to your child's MCH nurse, GP or paediatrician.

Closely watching a 'checklist' or calendar of developmental milestones may trouble parents if they think their child is not developing normally. At the same time, however, milestones can help to identify a child who needs a more detailed check-up.

Play

Play for babies from seven to eight weeks consists of tummy time and back time. It is so important to put your baby on a mat on the floor between feeds. This allows him to not only use some energy but also wake up and have a stretch after sucking on one breast. You can then rewrap him so he's ready to suck on the other side.

So many mums feed the baby on only one breast and, as the baby is wrapped, he may fall asleep and his mum thinks he is ready for bed. When you put the baby down to bed he wakes up in five minutes, you are then confused as he looked sleepy but once you put him into his cot he woke up. This can begin a cycle of rocking and trying to resettle a baby, but I have a simple way to help you and your baby. You actually have to drive this yourself by wrapping, unwrapping, putting him on the floor to play, then rewrapping and feeding.

A typical feed during the day would go like this:

- Pick up the baby when he is crying and ready for a feed. He should already be wrapped for sleep, so put him on the left breast, for example. Let him feed. When he has stopped sucking strongly, take him off even if he is asleep, unwrap him and give him some tummy time by putting him on his tummy next to you on the couch or on a rug on the floor.

- You can then massage his back gently, which will also help him burp. He will lift his head from one side to the other, looking for more food. In the early days he will only cope with a few minutes on his tummy, but that's okay because you will be doing it frequently during the day. Do *not* do this overnight: overnight it's feed and then back to sleep.

- Once he's had a few minutes' tummy time, turn him onto his back and change his nappy, then rewrap him and put him on the other breast to feed. He will be awake and ready to suck hard again. Once you've finished the second side you can actually unwrap and repeat the process. So it's feed, play, feed, play, feed then sleep.

Every baby is different, and some babies may need four to five or six feed-and-play cycles before they go back to sleep. If you put a baby down to bed and he wakes up within five minutes, he is either hungry or he needs more playtime. So you pick your baby up and go through the cycle again.

If you feed your baby on only one side, then put him to bed thinking he's had enough to drink because he's gone to sleep, you'll probably need to resettle him with either a dummy or soothing. This will not only make you feel anxious, but you'll underfeed your baby. If your baby is crying, feed him. In these first few weeks, babies want to feed to regain lost weight after birth, and you will not believe how much they need to feed. In fact, you will wonder how you ever left the house to go to work! Babies take up so much time, with feeding, changing nappies, holding them and just looking at how beautiful they are.

Sleep

All babies are different. Every day is different. So you can't compare your baby to anyone else's, or even to a sibling. Many mums say to me, 'My first child didn't do this.' I always say, 'Think about your own siblings. Are you all alike?' After a bit of a chuckle they realise their baby is a new person. Every day is different: one day you feel as if you have everything organised, the baby is feeding and sleeping beautifully and you think to yourself, 'I finally nailed it!' But the next day all hell breaks loose. No two days are the same and I encourage you to just respond to your baby on that day in that moment. Doing so will take a lot of pressure off you.

As far as sleeping goes, again, some babies seriously feed, sleep, feed, sleep, feed, sleep all day and all night. It's not that common but if your baby does this, celebrate and enjoy. Other babies are more demanding and that's just how it is;

you need to live in the moment and respond to your baby by feeding him and holding or carrying him around, and when he sleeps it's a bonus. Of course, some babies have reflux (see pages 58–60). Babies with reflux really don't sleep much at all and you need to hold them upright most of the day.

Your baby's overnight sleep really won't settle until he's about five to six weeks old. After his bath I would expect a five- or six-week-old baby to sleep from about 10.30 pm to 2 or 3 am. When he wakes up, feed him on one side, then change his nappy and feed him on the other side. Finish with a big cuddle and lots of kisses before putting him back to bed. In these early weeks your baby may have a bowel action overnight so you need to change his nappy. As the weeks go by he will have fewer bowel actions and if he doesn't have a poo overnight, you don't need to change his nappy at that feed. If a baby is sleeping well overnight—and I mean three to four hours after his bath—I would expect him to have a few small sleeps until 6 or 7 am.

As the weeks go by, once he's up in the morning, you need to encourage your baby to be awake more, feed more and play more. A lot of parents are afraid to change the routine they established in the early weeks, but the baby is changing every day—the routine has to change to suit his changing growth and development. And when you stick to a now outmoded routine, you're trying to get a baby to sleep who wants to stay awake and play and feed. This causes mothers great anxiety. You should encourage your baby to follow the feed, play, feed, play, feed, play routine until he's ready to sleep. Don't go by the clock to feed your baby; respond to his needs—that is, if he's crying, feed him. Once you've fed him and put him down on the floor to play and he starts to cry or is unsettled, pick him up and feed him again. Do that on repeat until the baby is tired and not only goes to sleep but also stays asleep.

If your seven- or eight-week-old baby isn't sleeping, you need sensible and practical advice; gimmicky methods and fads do not work. Many books by untrained so-called 'sleep gurus' try to teach parenting by using different 'tricks' to get babies to sleep. Some parents with three- or four-day-old babies (still in hospital) are taught by professionals to 'shush into your baby's ear and this will soothe them'. I can tell you without question that this is wrong. Babies need food, and plenty of it.

Your baby is not capable of sleeping through the night until he is old enough and has enough weight on him—usually well over six months. In the early days and weeks his brain is growing so quickly and he needs lots and lots of milk to help him grow. It takes time. Be patient.

The community can make it hard for women if their baby doesn't sleep 'through the night'; it's supposed to indicate that they are bad or incompetent mothers. There are waiting lists for 'sleep schools', and it's becoming a rite of passage for a mother to attend one. We need to take the stress and pressure off young families, and support and educate them to be patient with their little babies.

For your baby to sleep—seven key points

1. **The baby** Your baby is an individual. He will not sleep, eat, develop, play, talk, laugh, love like your friend's baby, your sister's baby, your neighbour's baby or even your other children. In the beginning, your baby will get days and nights mixed up; this is normal. Your baby cannot sleep all day then sleep all night. He needs a huge amount of feeding in the first six months to grow. I would expect a newborn baby in the first six weeks to be feeding every three to four hours during the day and, at the most, to sleep four to five hours after midnight.

2. **A routine** The BBB routine is not possible until the baby weighs at least 7 to 8 kilograms or is about three to four months old. The BBB routine is for night-time, while daytime is often two to three small sleeps of 45 minutes. I advise all my new mums and dads to start my bath, bottle and bed routine from the first day home from hospital (for an overview of the BBB method, see *TFSW*, pages 129–32). It is the first step towards getting your baby to sleep. One of the biggest traps new parents fall into is bathing a newborn baby at 6 pm every night, which is far too early for a new baby.

3. **Reflux** If your baby has gastric reflux he will not sleep much at all until the diagnosis and treatment is in place.

A baby with gastric reflux can be diagnosed at two to three weeks after birth: when he lies down he squirms, arches his back, screams and cries, and is only happy if he is feeding or being held upright. If any adult has suffered from reflux they will understand how uncomfortable the baby is, and why he can be labelled as 'difficult'. (For more information on gastric reflux, see pages 58–60)

4. **Wrapping** Babies need to be wrapped in large, light muslin wraps from birth for all feeding and sleeping. I invented a way of wrapping new babies that is safe and secure, and babies *love* it. Many years ago babies slept on their tummies, but with all the evidence of what causes SIDS, we know it is safer for babies to sleep on their backs. Once we started putting unwrapped babies on their backs to sleep, they found it difficult as the Moro reflex, one of the newborn's primitive reflexes that makes him startle and thrust up his arms, is very active and disturbing if they are on their backs. Wrapping the baby makes him feel as if he is back in the womb, safe and calm.

5. **Cath's Wrap** (see pages 33–35) My method of wrapping ensures the baby is wrapped with hands and arms bent up (as every baby loves to sleep like this) and their hips and legs are flexed and capable of full movement. It has been proven that a baby whose arms are wrapped by his

sides will fight the wrap, ending up with his arms out and scratching his face. It has also been proven that wrapping a baby's legs straight so he can't flex his hips is detrimental. Wrapping is the key to good feeding and sleeping.

6. **Food** Babies need to be fed, end of story! Breastfeed your baby. From side to side, hour to hour . . . keep going. Your baby will go to sleep when he has had enough to eat and not before. You cannot successfully rock, shush, pat your baby to sleep or put a dummy in his mouth and expect him to go to sleep. You can nurse a screaming baby all night but in the end he needs food. If you don't have enough breast milk, give your baby some formula. Don't sit and pump and pump and pump your milk—if your baby is hungry, feed him. Currently there's a worrying scare campaign against formula but it's food made specially for babies.

7. **Feed your baby to sleep** It's not a crime! Wrap your baby and feed him to sleep. What is more natural than to feed your baby until he is sound asleep and is put to bed calm and fed? Another scare campaign is that if you feed your baby to sleep he will never sleep alone. There is nothing wrong with keeping your newborn baby close, and again I ask the question—what is the alternative? Letting him scream to sleep?

Night-time routine

By the time the baby is eight weeks old he can be potentially sleeping five to six hours overnight. I would still be doing the BBB at 10 pm and not be tempted to bring the bath any earlier at this stage. I get lots of parents very eager to change the bath time and change the routine, to do it earlier, but it always fails. Please be patient and let the baby put on extra weight and grow a little older before doing this. There is no hurry.

We went to see Cath when our baby was only 10 days old. She explained the BBB routine to us and within a few nights we were in a perfect routine. My husband did the bath and I went to bed and our son slept four hours as Cath had told us he would. But soon, we let too many other voices get into our heads. The MCH nurse said he was going to bed 'far too late'; my parents said 'he won't grow if he doesn't sleep during the day'; other friends said 'we've never heard of babies being bathed at 10 pm' and on it went. We caved. By the time our Tom was eight weeks old we had him bathed by 6 pm, in bed by 7 pm and me crying from 7.30 to 9.30 pm trying to settle him to sleep. It had turned into a nightmare. I picked up *The First Six Weeks* again and told my husband we needed to see Cath. We made an appointment and, seriously, it was a miracle. Cath explained that Tom was just not ready to go to bed at 6 pm, that he needed more tummy time and feeding from 6 to 9 pm each night, before a bath. Then he should sleep about five hours. He did exactly that and has slept every night since.

— JIMMY & NATALIE

The most important thing is to respond to *your* baby. You will know if your baby needs to go to bed earlier and the BBB needs to be done earlier. But only bring the bath back by half-hour increments as he won't cope with any more dramatic changes to the bath and bedtime routine. The slower you move bath time the better his sleep will be. And once you get the baby sleeping well overnight you really don't want to do anything that is going to change his sleep. Two things will change his sleep—one is playtime during the awake times and the other is putting him to bed far too early when he is too young and his weight is not above 8 kilograms.

At seven to eight weeks the night-time usually consists of only one feed time. By this time the baby is very efficient and feed time is usually all done within half an hour. As the baby doesn't have a dirty nappy overnight it isn't necessary to change his nappy—feed on both breasts and put him back to bed.

Daytime routine

At eight weeks the daytime is all about feeding and playing, feeding and playing. Sleeping is secondary. You will find your baby has three or four, 30-minute long sleeps during the day, not long stretches. This is fine and it is all they can cope with. Trying to get a baby to sleep more causes a mum *so* much anxiety. I know other books and professionals say that babies need two to three hours of sleep during the day but when are they going to feed? Babies need to be awake to feed and play during the day and early evening and up until the late bath. That is when they are physically ready to sleep. It is much better for you as parents too, as you can get a solid sleep after midnight, which is when you need to have a deep sleep. You feel much more rested and recovered the next day.

Crying

Although crying is a normal part of your baby's development, when a seven- to eight-week-old baby cries it is for a good reason. At this age, crying can be a sign that your baby is getting sick. It is good to note here that when your baby changes behaviour at any stage he may be getting a cold or gastro. When a baby is getting a cold he will feel unwell a few days before he shows signs of a runny nose or a temperature.

Often that is when a baby is crying for what you think is 'no reason'. I advise if you feed a baby and he is not 'back to normal' and is still crying, then give him some paracetamol and see if in 30 minutes it has made any change to his crying. Keep an eye on him and, if necessary, have him checked by your GP.

Here are some other tips for dealing with a crying baby:

- Check if he has a wet or dirty nappy.
- See if a dummy comforts him after a feed.
- Bath him (it doesn't matter how many baths you give him a day, as long as it helps break the crying cycle).
- Hold him upright as much as you can (use a baby carrier, so you can hold him close while you do other things).
- Have him checked by your paediatrician, GP or MCH nurse in case he is unwell—for example, with gastric reflux (see pages 58–60).
- If you're feeling angry and anxious at all the crying, put your baby safely in his cot and leave the room for a few minutes to regroup before you pick him up again.
- Let your partner know how you're feeling and agree on some simple routines to give you some time out. For example, when your partner comes home from work, have a relaxing bath, or get out of the house for a walk.

One of the hardest issues to deal with is when your child is unwell. It's easy to overreact and, sometimes, you don't know if your reaction is warranted or not. Stay calm, getting yourself worked up doesn't help. Follow your gut. If you're hesitating about seeking professional advice, just do it. It won't hurt. I make bookings with my doctor online, so I can do it at any time, and knowing I have a booking the next day is comforting. Don't be shy about Panadol—use it. It's a fantastic resource. Also get a digital thermometer—it's such a relief to see when your baby's temperature goes down.

— SAM

Being a parent is a 24-hour job and you'll have great days and not so great days. As soon as you give birth, your life changes—you are responsible for a little baby and this can be confronting. It's also the best time of your life! Enjoy every day. Be patient.

7

Two to four months

I am over eight weeks old, and I've come a long way in such a short time. I can see you clearly and I love you more than anything in the world (other than milk). I hope you enjoy my loving smiles. Be patient with me as I learn to sleep longer, I will get there . . . I'm still a little baby!

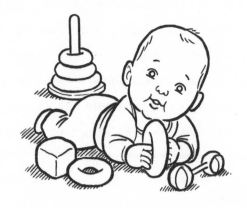

Feeding your baby

Milk

During this period your baby will grow and develop a lot, so he needs a lot of food—and by food, I mean milk. His intake will increase as he grows from two to four months, in line with his increased activity. He will have a very good drink first thing in the morning.

If you are breastfeeding, your supply will be well and truly established by now, and the initial feeling of fullness in your breasts after birth will have settled. Even though your breasts may feel soft and 'normal', you will still be lactating. Remember that the milk supply is made by your brain triggering oxytocin, a hormone that makes your breasts eject the milk when the baby sucks, so that is why your breasts may feel softer, and 'normal'. This doesn't mean that your milk supply has 'gone' or 'dried up'. Mother Nature is very smart—she wants a woman's body to keep lactating (even though we all lactate differently), so for your lactation to cease, either you have to actively wean your baby off your breast or your baby—for many reasons—stops attaching to your breast.

Development

Developmental and behavioural check-ups are an important aspect of childhood health care. Not only do they give parents a good idea of their child's development and behaviour, they also help identify any developmental or behavioural delays and problems as early as possible. These problems are reasonably common, but research demonstrates that early identification and, consequently, early intervention improves both short- and long-term outcomes.

In general, your baby's developmental skills can be organised into four areas:

- gross motor (that is, core and large muscle) movements
- fine motor (that is, hand and smaller muscle) movements
- communication (that is, expressive verbal and non-verbal language and receptive language)
- socialisation.

In the following table you'll find some of the milestones that can be expected in the above areas at two months (and this is updated in the following chapters). A key aspect of these milestones, and one that I try to emphasise to parents—especially those who are worried about their child's development—is to not consider a milestone in isolation. I think it is important to look at what else your baby is doing at that particular age, as well as whether he has made developmental progress at a steady rate leading up to that point; if he has, it can often be reassuring.

Two months

Gross motor	Fine motor
• Starting to hold head up when lying on tummy	• Smoother arm and leg movements • Hands unfisted some of the time • Holding hands together

Social	Communication
• Smiles at people • Follows faces • Visually tracks large, highly contrasting objects • Turns head towards sounds • Startles in response to loud noises	• Cooes or makes gurgling sounds • Responds to voices

Play

Food + Play = Sleep

Community professionals traditionally teach 'feed, play, sleep' but, for several reasons, it often doesn't work. In practice, you need to modify this for every baby. Think about yourself—if you had breakfast, went to work and then came home and went to bed with nothing to eat or drink, that would be the 'feed, play, sleep' model that is currently promoted. In reality, you get up, have breakfast, go to work, have morning tea, do more work, have lunch, do more work, have afternoon tea, come home, have dinner, and then you go to bed.

A baby, on the other hand, has to go to bed both well fed (kilojoules in) and tired (energy out). A hungry baby won't go to sleep, and a baby who has not played enough will not be sufficiently tired to sleep. As the baby gets older, he must spend more and more time playing. That play should happen with the baby flat on the floor—not in a swinging chair or seat or even sitting on the floor. This does not use up enough of your baby's energy to tire him.

He needs a balance—an increase in food requires an increase in activity, otherwise he is not going to sleep when you want him to; and you will be anxious, exhausted and wondering why your baby is not sleeping! It's not good for anyone.

My 'feed, play, feed, play, feed, play' method works brilliantly!

When he gets tired and grisly, rather than put him to bed, give him a feed on one breast, or give him a bottle. Then put him back down onto the floor for some more floor time. Think about it—if you feed your baby then let him play for an hour or so and then put him down to bed, nine times out of ten he will not go to sleep. Why? He is hungry because he has had a lot of play but not enough milk *or* he's had milk but not enough play.

I remember when Leo, our first, was two weeks old. It was Christmas Day and Cath was over at our place. After a while she said, 'Give me Leo, he needs to be on the floor! He needs to burn energy, then he will feed better and sleep better.' It was like a revelation to me!! In my sleep-deprived state, living in the whole new overwhelming world of babies, I actually don't think in his two short weeks I'd let his feet touch the ground, literally!

We were taught by Cath that babies don't need any gadgets/seats/bouncers; they learn everything just by being on the floor. So that's what we did. Tummy time and floor time every day from then on with Leo, and from day 1 with Anna and Georgie, our next two.

Very quickly their necks get strong, they learn to roll, pivot, get up on their hands and knees and rock, crawl and walk—it is absolutely amazing to watch the progressive development.

It's staggering just how much 'stuff' there is out there for babies and how much people think they need; I would have thought the same had it not been for Cath. Before having Leo I was kindly given a bouncer. After having him on the floor all the time, one day I thought maybe I should try this bouncer—he didn't enjoy the restriction of it, so we didn't use it and he was much happier on the floor.

We learnt to politely decline if friends offered these things they didn't need anymore. They may be handy for parents who want to keep their kids still for a minute while they do what they need to, but in the long run they really don't help with development.

All of our babies have hit their milestones by the book—they all have rolled by three to four months, crawled by six to seven months and walked by 11 months. My youngest is now eight months, pulling herself up all the time and starting to cruise around the furniture.

People often comment that our children were early at hitting these milestones, but Cath has reassured me it's due to them having freedom on the floor. I have just let them do what they should be doing. The development of a baby in their first year is astounding; we just have to let them do it.

— KYLIE

Play, feed, play routine when you're out

Of course, you don't want to stay at home all day, so feed your baby before you go out. If you're on foot, the baby can have his playtime in the pram. When he becomes grizzly he can have another feed, then go back into the pram to lie flat for a play. Then give him another feed when he needs it.

Tummy time

When a baby is on his tummy, he has to work hard, use his muscles and, most importantly, start his progressive development. He has to push up, turn his neck from side to side, instinctively looking for a nipple or food source. He will also turn towards the sound of your voice, look at noisy, colourful objects, and move around a bit to listen to various sounds. So it's important for the development of your baby's upper-body strength to let him spend some time on his tummy from day 1!

This ultimately helps your baby progressively develop and learn to push up, roll over, sit up, crawl, pull himself up to cruise the furniture, then stand and, ultimately, walk. Tummy time also reduces the chance of your baby developing a flat spot on his head—called plagiocephaly or flat head syndrome (see pages 54–55)—from spending too much time on his back: the soft bones of the skull can be forced flat if he stays on his back during playtime on the floor. As all babies are now put down to sleep on their backs, we need to ensure their daytime play is a combination of tummy time and back time.

As your baby gets older and stronger he will be capable of staying on his tummy for a longer period of time. If he starts to cry, turn him onto his back or pick him up . . . then try tummy time again.

The popular and best way for your baby to practise tummy time is on a clean and soft quilt on the floor. Use the same quilt or soft blanket each time so your baby knows it's play-time. Or try lying on the floor or bed yourself, then laying the baby on you, tummy to tummy. You will both love it, plus your baby can see you, hear your heartbeat and smell you.

Sleep

Sleep for a baby at this age is usually quite settled overnight, but he can be all over the place during the day. Don't panic. Babies cannot sleep all night and then sleep all day; they have to have their kilojoules (milk) at some stage. Plus, as I have already mentioned, they need play and lots of it.

Now your baby is two to four months old and is usually capable of sleeping six to seven hours overnight—that is, after the bath and bottle. The usual waking time for a baby at this age is 4 am. Do not try to resettle the baby at 4 am; feed him when he wakes and put him back to bed for another few hours' sleep. At this time of night your breasts should be nice and full, and you'll find it's a very quick and efficient feed. I encourage you to feed one side, unwrap the baby, change his nappy, rewrap him, then feed on the other side.

Always stay with your baby for an extra for 10 to 20 minutes after the feed, holding him over your shoulder while you gently rub his back—not to burp him, just for that close comfort and love overnight. Believe me, these days go very quickly—one day you may look longingly back at these beautiful night-time moments together! After the 4 am feed, your baby will often settle and sleep till about 7 am.

What a typical day and night might look like

During the daytime, especially if your baby is sleeping well at night, he won't usually sleep much during the day. He can't do both—sleep day and night—unless he's sick. You're not going to have a perfect daytime routine for a baby at this age, it will happen, but not just yet.

Sleeping well both at night and during the day doesn't happen until the baby is about six or seven months, when he is involved in increased activity (rolling, active on tummy and back, and crawling). Your baby will eventually sleep for longer periods but, like all things, it takes time. Be patient.

Below is a *guide only*—no two babies are the same, so if your baby sleeps longer during the day, that's okay. If your baby doesn't sleep much during the day and is well, that's okay too.

A baby between two and four months should be feeding and playing frequently in the *morning* with maybe a 30- to 45-minute nap at lunchtime. Then, after lunch, he should be feeding and playing frequently in the *afternoon* again, with another 30- to 60- minute sleep.

I often find with a baby at this age that it's good to give him a bottle of formula at 5 pm to get him through to the 10 pm bath. Babies are so clever—they know by now that night-time is sleep time and to sleep they need lots of milk. They will put on more weight and that's how they start to sleep longer hours overnight.

So from 6 to 9.30 pm it's feed, play, feed, play, feed, play, feed, play and maybe a nap of 30 minutes here and there, just to tide him over to bedtime after the bath.

Once 9.30 pm comes, follow my BBB routine—prepare the bath so your partner can bath your baby, give him a bottle of formula and put him to bed. Hopefully you can go to bed by 9 o'clock to get some well-earned sleep.

Bringing back the bath time

As your baby approaches four months of age and his weight increases to about 7 kilograms, you will find that he will need to have his bath earlier—he will be showing signs of tiredness and isn't capable of staying awake until the 10 o'clock bath. So bring the bath back in small increments of half an hour—from 10 pm to 9.30 pm, then to 8.30 pm, then 8 pm. Don't hurry this process as we don't want to interrupt the wonderful sleep after midnight for both you and your baby.

It's best to continue keeping the baby up from 6 to 9 pm, feeding and playing, feeding and playing. At this stage you're looking at giving him a bath at around 9 pm. Continue to wrap him, and as he is capable of taking more formula, offer him what he needs. He may be drinking up to 120 to 150 ml after the bath by this stage.

If he doesn't settle straight away he is not ready to sleep. Rather than anxiously patting him to get him to sleep, get him out of bed, unwrap him, give him some tummy time, massage his back, then give him some back time, and change his nappy, rewrap him, and offer him another bottle of formula. If your baby doesn't settle by about 10 pm, don't panic: at this age and weight he is capable of sleeping easily through to 4 am.

Hair loss

Hair growth is very common during pregnancy, and some women with very curly hair notice that their hair becomes straight. On the other hand, hair loss three months after the birth is very common, and what's so distressing is that your hair can fall out in clumps. Most women's hair regrows after about six months to 12 months. If you have an issue with extreme hair loss it might be best to check with your doctor and have some blood tests done.

When you have your first baby it is perfectly normal to feel at some stage like you can't cope, but your confidence will grow with the baby. No one can learn your job in one day so don't expect to be an expert parent instantly. Be patient with yourself, respond to your baby's needs and keep life simple. Food. Love. Warmth.

8

Four to six months

I'm learning so much now I'm over four months old. I'm visually insatiable and interested in the world around me. I dribble a lot. I put everything in my mouth—even my toes—because I can! I love you, and I love simple games. Keep talking to me—that's how I'm going to learn. Keep me playing on the floor, that's how I will learn to roll!

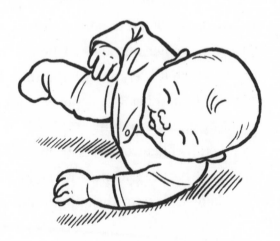

Feeding your baby

Breast milk

From four to six months your baby's milk intake will continue to increase. Your breastfeeding is well and truly established by now, but you may find that your baby only sucks for a short period during each feed. Babies often fuss at the breast at this age, usually because they are easily distracted. Try not to force him to feed and if he fusses consistently, take him off the breast and onto the floor to play. Then pick him up and try him again. Usually babies then knuckle down and have a very effective and efficient feeding session.

Professionals use phrases like 'your baby is snacking' when the baby is having shorter and frequent breastfeeds. The phrase is used to imply you are doing something wrong. Many mothers are at a loss to know what to do when this happens. It's not a problem. We may snack as adults, but babies feed. Every time they are on the breast or taking a bottle, it's a feed. As I keep saying, your baby really knows when he is hungry, so trust him (even though it's very annoying at times). As long as he is gaining weight and has wet nappies at every nappy change, he is getting enough to drink.

Don't worry if you feel like your breasts are soft and your milk has depleted—it hasn't. Lactation is the hardest thing to get rid of. Your body is lactating beautifully and your baby is efficiently drinking enough milk, exactly what he needs for the day.

Formula

If you are formula feeding, your baby may be drinking well over 1 litre of formula a day. Again, every baby is different: some babies will have more bottles with less formula in each one, while others will have five to six bottles a day with 180 to 210 ml per feed. Always respond to your baby's needs. Don't stretch out his feeds, as he needs all the food he asks for. I like to write down the amount the baby has each day and then you know how much he is having.

Your baby may be easily distracted during feeds at this age—see above under 'Breast milk' for more information.

Mixed feeding

If you are breastfeeding and topping up with formula, I encourage you to always breastfeed both sides first. Then, when your baby requires a top-up, offer him what he needs. Never reduce your baby's milk intake or stretch out a feed. Mother Nature has hardwired him to live, and the only way he lives is by drinking milk and gaining weight. And that's how a baby gets to sleep longer overnight. So keep feeding. It's all about food and weight gain!

What happens if my baby wants to feed all day?

If your baby is feeding constantly at this age, he obviously requires extra kilojoules. There are two things to consider:

- If he is constantly sucking at the breast and not gaining weight, he needs some extra formula.
- If he wants to sit on your lap and be held all day, that's different. It's usually a behavioural issue, especially if he is of a good weight. He needs more play.

So, if your baby needs extra kilojoules and you find that he is actually on the breast for a long time, you need to top up with some formula maybe once or twice a day. Always offer the breast, and try not to use a dummy, as all this will do is allow him to suck without getting any food (kilojoules).

If his crying is a behavioural issue and he's wanting to be held, that's okay—that's what babies do at this age—as long as you are happy to hold him. At this age babies can develop a form of 'fear of strangers' and become *very* attached to their parents. It's so important in the early parenting of babies to keep them very close, so don't dismiss this behaviour in your baby as whingeing, or worry that you're not being tough enough.

Also, remember that babies tend to cling to you more when they're very tired, teething, unwell or after an immunisation. If your baby has a temperature or he's had an immunisation in the past 24 hours, you can give him some paracetamol, which should settle him. If you see a change in him within 20 minutes you know that he has been in some discomfort.

If your baby is tired, obviously you need to address his sleeping routine. If he doesn't sleep well at night, he will tend to be very cranky during the day. That's why I like to have babies sleeping well overnight so they are happier during the day (even though they may not sleep long hours in the daytime).

Introducing solids

Ideally, a baby has breast milk or formula only for the first six months, then they should be slowly introduced to solids.

Learning to eat is a big milestone for your baby, and I want it to be free of anxiety for both of you. There is absolutely no need to rush into feeding your baby solids. There seems to be a competition in the community and pressure from health professionals to have your baby eating solids early. There are few things in life that are inevitable, but one of them is that your child will eventually eat solid food. There is nothing to be gained by pressuring your baby to eat—forcing food on him, following him around with a spoon, turning the television on to distract him while you try to feed him or making 30 different meals that you think your child might like.

Let. It. Go.

I'm sorry to say that most issues with feeding solids to babies come from the mother. Often she is under a lot of pressure from *her* mother and also, as I said before, from professionals. How and when you introduce your baby to solids is important because it can affect your child for the rest of his life. That's how serious I am about introducing your child to solids at the right time and keeping it stress-free, anxiety-free and relaxed!

Your baby needs to be ready—to eat, to swallow, to chew, to use a spoon, to open his mouth, and to try new tastes and textures. If we force a certain behaviour onto a child he will react in a negative way, and that reaction will become a habit and, unfortunately, a bad one. How many second and third children in a family have an issue with eating? Zero. It's because their mother has no time for fussing around, playing aeroplanes, or following the baby with a last spoonful of mixed vegetables to ensure the child finishes his food. By the time she's had her second, third and fourth baby, the mum is so organised and relaxed she's just happy to get through the day! And, of course, the baby eats easily.

When a baby dribbles it's not because he's teething but because he has a lot of sputum in his mouth he can't swallow. So, while he's playing, concentrating or sitting in the pram, he sits with his mouth open and drools. The extended family will tell you that dribbling means he's starting to get teeth. Developmentally, however, he needs to be able to move this sputum around his mouth and swallow before he can cope with eating. Sometimes a baby may not be ready to eat solid food until he is six or seven months old.

There is always an exception to the rule, and some babies just open their mouth at six months and off they go, eating everything that's put in front of them. Their parents now think they have the perfect child. If you have a 'fussy eater'—when your child takes one taste of vegetables and spits it out—you need to slow down, back off, and start again in a few days or weeks. There is no hurry. Be patient.

Most importantly, although we know we shouldn't compare our child with others, we can't help looking at other people's children and thinking to ourselves, 'My child isn't doing that', and for some reason we feel very guilty. It's really important to be your own self and your own parent with your child; there is no need to feel guilty when you love and care for your child. It's all about surviving each day with a happy and healthy baby who has happy and healthy parents.

To eat solids, babies need to be ready, sitting up confidently and looking interested. This doesn't mean watching you eating your dinner. Babies tend to be visually excited by colour and movement and will watch when you eat and move your hand from your plate to your mouth. They don't understand that you are eating food. And it doesn't mean they are ready for solids. It's true that some babies are sensitive and take longer to eat well—for example, premature babies, or babies who have had reflux or vomited frequently in the early weeks may have issues with eating solid food. Wait until your baby is ready. The milk he's having is fine; there is no need to feel anxious or make your baby anxious and end up with a child with a long-term feeding aversion.

I had my baby girl at 38 weeks by caesarean section. She weighed 2.8 kilograms. I tried to breastfeed in hospital and found the pressure to do so from the midwives just overwhelming. It may be I was just very anxious as a first-time mum. My family were very supportive and by the time we got home I was giving her some formula, breastfeeding a few times and also offering some expressed breast milk. After six long weeks my husband and I finally decided to put our daughter on formula. The extreme pressure from the community and the hospital, and comparing my baby to other babies really made me very anxious.

I must say here that neither my husband nor I are very tall people. When I went to the MCH service I kept being told that my baby should take at least 120 ml in each bottle. She could only manage 60 ml but the professional told us we had to push her. In hindsight, I really felt we force-fed her that extra 60 ml. So, after a lot of feeds she vomited the extra 60 ml; sometimes it looked like she'd thrown up the whole feed.

By three months our daughter was not taking much formula and had only had a small weight gain. There was so much pressure. We took her to nearly every emergency department to be checked out; they threatened to put a tube down her nose into her stomach if she became dehydrated.

While I was pregnant, my husband and I had met Cath at a pregnancy expo. When our daughter was nine months old, I remembered her and asked for a phone consultation.

We told her our story and she listened. One thing she wanted to see was a photo of our daughter. The first thing she said to us was, 'This baby is not sick.' It was such a relief to hear 'your baby will be fine' from a true professional. We still had a battle in front of us but Cath's reassurance was tremendous; she was on our side.

Cath kept saying, 'She will eat, she will drink, it will happen, but you must be patient.' We learnt that our daughter had a severe feeding aversion because we force-fed her, and all because we thought we were doing the right thing, as the professionals told us she needed a certain amount of milk in each bottle.

We went to speech pathologists, paediatricians and other specialists and we were given a variety of reasons why our daughter wasn't drinking. In hindsight, she just had a tiny frame; at three years old she still is quite petite.

To make a long story short, our daughter basically lived on milk for up to 18 months. Introducing solids was a nightmare as she would chew and keep the food in her mouth until I removed it. She ate some foods with a soft texture, and no chewing or swallowing took place. She was on the follow-on milk (milk for babies after they are 12 months old), so she was getting enough kilojoules.

I can't say she is 100 per cent perfect with her eating now, but she does eat and has made huge progress. Subsequently, I had another child, and Cath and I determined that he was not going to have the same issues. We bottle-fed him straight away and it has been so much easier than with our daughter. But I still had anxiety because of the trauma we went through with our first child.

Our son was eating all his food puréed and I know I kept the food puréed because of my anxiety around food. I met with Cath before his first birthday and told her that he was having soft foods only. She encouraged me to slowly introduce him to thicker food. Literally, one day he was eating purée and then the next day he just ate a chop! I was ecstatic.

I would like to reach out to each and every one of you and encourage you to neither force your baby to drink or eat, nor compare the child with anyone else. When we looked at the percentiles for our daughter, she was in proportion, and still is. Cath was right—it took time, but she is eating now and she is the most adorable little girl.

The effect of our daughter's feeding aversion not only on her but also on us and our extended families was immense. Everyone has a cure, and everyone has advice. I knew she wasn't sick, so it was the pressure of the feeding aversion that really made me feel very anxious. I'm grateful I have two healthy and happy children who will never be six feet tall.

— JENNY

How do you know when to introduce solids?
Over the years, professional opinion on when to introduce solids has varied; some professionals advocate introducing solids at four months. The physical characteristics that allow for the introduction of solid foods between the ages of four and six months include:

- the disappearance of the extrusion reflex (see below), which occurs at around four months, enabling the baby to move food to the back of his mouth and swallow safely
- more developed head control, which enables the baby to swallow more easily when sitting
- your baby sticking his tongue in and out when you start to feed him solids.

The extrusion reflex

This reflex—to push anything hard away from his mouth—is a primitive but normal one your baby was born with. Mother Nature has hardwired him to protect himself from hard and possibly dangerous objects or food that he is not yet able to chew and swallow. It's not that he doesn't like food; it's all about sucking at this stage of his life. When the extrusion reflex disappears in a healthy baby, he is able to move food to the back of his mouth and swallow safely. This is when your baby is ready for solids.

Over time, a child's ability to manage the change in textures—from liquids to solids—develops. When deciding whether to introduce your baby to solids, consider his readiness for, and interest in, food. Some babies will be interested in food earlier than others—even in the same family you may have each child start eating food at a different age. You need to take into account your baby's age, weight and developmental progress, so don't worry if your mother or mother-in-law is keen to introduce her grandchild to solids.

For a baby, learning to eat requires time, patience and a variety of food, and no anxiety for either mother or baby. Feeding aversion can start early if you force your baby to take solid food. It's the last thing you need. So if your baby refuses food one day, leave it for a few days, then start over again. Your baby will eat, it will happen, but you need him to be ready.

Solid foods to start with

In your baby's first year, gradually introduce him to a variety of foods in small amounts, one at a time, from each of these food groups: cereals, dairy, meat, poultry, fish, fruit and vegetables. Keep it simple, soft, clean and fresh. Your baby does not need a gourmet menu but it is good to make sure he has no allergic reactions to certain foods (see pages 171–72).

Offer only one food at a time. Start with a teaspoon of food and gradually increase the amount over the following days and weeks. An iron-enriched infant cereal, such as rice cereal, is an ideal food to begin with. At breakfast, mix a teaspoon of cereal with some breast milk or formula, which provides the baby with added kilojoules. He may react to the cereal with some funny faces, as the taste and texture are both new to him. If he refuses the first time, try again the next day. Take your time and don't hurry, as meal times are meant to be relaxing and stress-free.

Once the baby has had rice cereal for a few days, introduce some stewed apples at lunchtime. Continue this for another few days. Then introduce some mashed sweet potato at dinnertime. So now you have a menu plan:

- rice cereal for breakfast
- stewed apples for lunch
- mashed sweet potato for dinner.

As the days and weeks go by, you'll add new foods. Again, with each new food, start with a teaspoon and gradually increase the amount over the following days and weeks. Only offer one food at a time, as that is how we eliminate any foods to which the baby is allergic.

Foods not to give a baby under 12 months

- It is not necessary to add any sugar or salt to your baby's food, just to suit your taste as an adult.
- Fast foods, foods high in sugar and fat, and soft drinks and fruit juices, which are very high in sugar, are not suitable for a growing child.
- Do not give him small, hard foods, such as nuts and uncooked vegetables, due to the risk of inhalation and choking.
- It is not advisable to give honey to children under 12 months because of the potential risk of *Clostridium botulinum* (botulism).

Some general advice

- Offer your baby a range of textures—soft, puréed or runny to start, and then thicken as the baby gets older and can cope with thicker textures. Include different tastes, such as savoury, bitter, sour and sweet.
- Warm his food to start with, then change to cooler.
- Be prepared for the mess as your baby learns to eat—messy is good! He will learn table manners later.
- Offer your baby milk for thirst.
- Stay with your baby when he is eating and, where possible, sit him with the family at mealtimes so he can watch and learn feeding skills.
- When your baby starts eating foods other than milk, expect to see a change in bowel habits (and smell).

Development

Four months

Gross motor	Fine motor
• Good head control • Sits with support • Lifting head to 90 degrees while on tummy • Rests on elbows/forearms while lying on tummy • Pushes down on surface with legs while being held upright • Tries to roll in one direction	• Recognises familiar faces and starts to interact more with others • Smiles and laughs • Follows moving objects with his eyes from side to side and across a room

Social	Communication
• Reaches out for objects	• Vocalises/babbles to get attention, have his needs met and when spoken to
• Brings hands to mouth	
• Attempts to pick up objects with both hands	• Cries in different ways to show hunger, pain or tiredness
	• Looks at others when they speak

Play

Play is so important for your baby when he's between the ages of four and six months.

Most of the calls I get are about babies who have been doing the BBB routine and sleeping perfectly since they were born, but have hit four months and things have started to unravel (see 'Four-month sleep regression', page 166). When your baby is about this age, he needs to burn up a lot more energy.

Most mums fall into the same trap at this stage. It's a common theme when I do phone or Skype consultations—mums tell me, 'I tried sitting my baby up and he's really happy and he loves playing with his toys, but he's stopped sleeping at night-time.' What's happening is that while the baby is getting lots of milk, he's just sitting, not using up any energy.

The same applies to putting the baby in a walker, any plastic sitting container, or a bouncy seat that hangs from a doorframe—these gadgets do not let the baby play or use his energy. My advice is get rid of them all and go on putting the baby on a lovely quilt on the floor so he has the freedom to move and play, making him hungry and tired—and that all equals sleep!

Daytime routine

Think of your day as being split into three sections—the morning, the afternoon and the early evening.

Once your day starts and you've changed your baby's nappy, offer him a drink of milk. Then it's time for play on the floor—tummy time, back time, tummy time, back time. And remember, don't be tempted to sit your baby up.

When he starts to protest or grizzle on the floor, offer him a drink then put him back down on the floor for more tummy time and playtime. Then repeat and repeat until he is tired and his time on the floor shortens. By this stage you'll know when he is not capable of any more play, so wrap him and give him a drink, then put him to bed.

Even if he sleeps for only 40 minutes or an hour, that's fine. He may sleep for two hours—that's fine too—but what I want to impress on you is that if the baby has small sleeps, it's really okay. He is not a cadet at boot camp, and your baby cannot do as he is told.

The word 'catnap' is often used to describe a baby's short sleep. Some mums think it's bad for their baby to have catnaps, but at this age they only sleep for short periods during the day— but frequently—and then they sleep for a longer stretch overnight.

You need to respond to his needs:

- if he is hungry, feed him
- if he is awake, let him play
- if he is tired, let him sleep
- when he wakes, feed him, then play, and so the day goes on.

Repeat that pattern in the *afternoon* and in the *early evening* until bath time.

Of course, you're not going to stay at home all day, and sometimes babies have their short naps in the car or in their pram—that's perfectly fine. Life has to go on, and you need to get out of the house and keep up your activities, run errands or see friends and family.

Evening routine

For the evening session prior to the bath, again, it is important to follow the repetitive feed, play, feed, play, sleep routine. You'll find that your baby will need to have his bath earlier. So keep bringing it back in small increments of half an hour—from 8 pm to 7.30 pm, then 7 pm, and so on.

Sleep

At this age your baby can be in a really good sleeping routine overnight but all over the place during the day. All I want is for babies to sleep a long stretch overnight. But they *can't* do that and then sleep all day.

So when your baby is this age you need to be patient and work on him sleeping well overnight, while expecting him to have three to four little naps during the day. Don't try to resettle a baby who's only had 40 to 45 minutes' sleep. That will only make both you and your baby unhappy, and then everyone in the household will become tense and you end up booking into sleep school—and really, it's totally unnecessary if you start your baby sleeping properly from day 1. Be patient. It takes time.

When your baby wakes from a 40-minute sleep, pick him up, change his nappy and give him a drink, then put him back down on the floor for a play. This is so important and I will talk more about it in regards to the four-month sleep regression (see page 166).

The BBB routine

So, basically you have a baby going to bed after the bath around 8 pm and, as he gets closer to six months, that will come closer to 6.30 pm. After the bath and breastfeed, hopefully the baby sleeps (still wrapped), till about 4 am. If your baby is sleeping overnight from the bath to 4 am, don't be in any hurry to move the bath to an earlier time—your baby will just wake up earlier—2 or 3 am—and, believe me, you don't want that!

I do encourage a dream feed at 10 pm at this age. Either you or your partner picks up your sleeping baby and offers him a bottle of formula or expressed breast milk in his sleep. Some babies can take up to 200 ml or more at this feed. After a cuddle over your shoulder and a burp, kiss your baby, tell him you love him and put him back into bed. The aim is to top him up with milk so he'll sleep through till about 4 am.

There is some controversy about giving a baby a bottle at night. You may wish to fully breastfeed your baby. But today I find both parents want to be involved with feeding the baby. When your partner gives your baby a bath and then a bottle at night, it creates a lovely bond between the two of them.

When the baby wakes again, you pick him up and either breastfeed him or, if you are formula feeding, give him a bottle. This should get him through to 6 or 7 am when your day starts. Change his nappy, offer him a drink of milk and then it's floor time—tummy time, back time, tummy time, back time—and remember, don't give into temptation and sit your baby up.

When he starts to protest or grizzle on the floor, he's telling you he needs to have a cuddle or a drink, so offer him a drink and then put him back down on the floor for more tummy time and playtime.

So repeat and repeat the play/feed cycle until he is tired and his time on the floor shortens. Wrap him up, give him a drink and then put him to bed.

Four-month sleep regression

Some babies are not moving enough. They are sitting in one spot, such as in prams and car seats, for far too long and this is interrupting sleep at night. This all happens around the age of four to five months. This new phenomenon has been labelled 'four-month sleep regression'. At the risk of sounding like a broken record, it's all to do with feeding and playing.

Think about yourself. If you ate breakfast in bed and just stayed there all day, reading a book or magazines, you wouldn't be tired at night and you'd have trouble sleeping properly. Part of our daily routine is not only to have a dietary intake but also be active throughout the day. Then when night-time comes, we are tired and we sleep. The same principle applies to babies!

If you feed your baby, and then just let him sit there—on the floor or in a bouncer or a jumper, or in anything that keeps him still—he is not using up his energy. This is why your baby's sleep starts to go downhill.

I see this constantly in my practice. All you have to do is get rid of the 'containers', as I call them. Feed your baby, then put him on the floor. Give him freedom to play, move and develop. Your baby will then be tired and want to sleep. It might seem like 'magic', but it's just common sense.

Enjoy feeding your baby
solids, and make mealtimes
a relaxing and pleasurable
experience. Try not to bring
your anxieties to the table.
Relax, talk to your baby and
help him love and enjoy
eating and food.

9

Six to eight months

Wow, I think I'm so clever—I know you do too as I can hear you telling Nana every day. Are you happy now I can sleep better for you overnight? I love the games you play with me, especially peekaboo—I could play that for hours. I know I'm on the move and keep you busy but I so enjoy our walks and talks together.

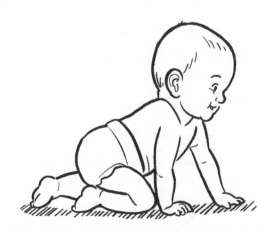

Feeding your baby

Milk

Breast milk or formula is still the primary food for a baby at this age; he still needs a lot of milk. I recommend introducing solid foods around six months, but not before four months.

If your baby is refusing solid food initially, stop for a few days to give the baby a break and then start again. Be patient. There's no hurry. A baby learning to eat needs time, patience, a variety of food and a relaxed mother. The last thing you need is a baby who develops an aversion to breastfeeding, taking a bottle or eating solid food. Feeding aversion can start early when mums are trying very hard to nearly force babies to either breastfeed, bottle feed or take solid food. If your baby is fussing and rejecting the breast, I suggest taking him off the breast, calming him down and then putting him on the floor for a bit of play. Then rewrap him and start again.

The last thing you should do is continuously try to put the baby on the breast, which will make both of you anxious. Most babies, when breastfed and taking a bottle once or twice a day, will continue to breastfeed long-term, and the mother's lactation will be perfect.

Solids

When your baby is six to seven months old, introduce minced red meats and minced chicken. At seven to eight months, give him small amounts of cow's milk in custard, yoghurt and on cereal.

Introducing foods that may cause allergies

In the early years, many children have common allergies to some foods, including—but not limited to—eggs, peanuts and dairy. It's advisable to introduce foods that may cause an allergic reaction before the baby turns one. If he has an allergic reaction, seek medical help (urgently if there is a severe reaction). Your GP may refer you to a paediatrician, who will then refer you to a specialist in allergies.

Egg and peanut allergies

Offering a baby peanuts and egg is important once your baby is more than six months of age. I am always very careful, even overcautious, when offering these foods to a baby, and I do it the old-fashioned way.

For peanuts, it's best to put a very small amount of smooth peanut butter on your clean little finger and place that on the inside of the baby's lip. If he is allergic, he will only have a local reaction, whereas if he swallows the peanut butter the inside of his mouth and throat could swell. That is really frightening! If there is no immediate allergic reaction, it is safe to say that he is not allergic to peanuts.

For egg—the first thing to offer is the yolk (the yellow part of the egg), which contains fewer allergens than egg white.

Cook a poached egg and, using your clean little finger, put a dot of the cooked yolk on the inside of your baby's lower lip. If there is any reaction, his lower lip will swell. Seek advice from your GP or paediatrician and don't offer him any more egg.

If your baby is okay with the yolk, the next day offer him half a teaspoon and allow him to swallow. As the days and weeks go by, offer him the full yolk.

The next thing to do is offer the egg white in exactly the same way as the yolk—dip your clean little finger into cooked egg white and put a small amount on your baby's inner lip. If you notice any swelling of the lips, eyes or face straight away, or soon after giving the egg white, or any new food, your baby could be having an allergic reaction. Always stop giving him that particular food and seek medical advice. If your baby is having a severe reaction, call an ambulance immediately. This is why you introduce one food at a time, so you know which food is causing the allergic reaction. It's rare for babies to have severe anaphylaxis (which is a sudden, widespread, potentially severe and life-threatening allergic reaction) but many babies have allergies to different foods.

I once looked after a lady who had made herself an egg for lunch. She washed her hands and then gave her baby, who was over six months, her regular meal. There must've been a trace of egg on her hand, as her baby's face came out in a bad rash. When tested, the baby certainly did have an allergy to egg. But when she was more than two years of age, she grew out of it.

Development

Six months

Gross motor	Fine motor
• Rolls over in both directions	• Reaches for and grasps objects
• Sits well with support, and starting to sit better without support	• Brings objects to his mouth
• Starts to support his own weight while standing	• Starts to pass objects from one hand to another
• Starts to bounce on his feet	
• Starts to push up with his hands and extended elbows when in the tummy position and pivoting	
• Tries to get up on his hands and knees	

Social	Communication
• Recognises familiar faces and is starting to identify strangers	• More babbling, with vowel sounds
• Enjoys playtime with others	• Takes turns making sounds with adult, and responds to sound by making sounds
• Responds to other people's emotions	
• Likes to look at himself in a mirror	• Starts to respond to his name, or momentarily stops to 'no'

Play

Until now your baby has basically stayed wherever you left him. Now he is mobile and should be rolling, doing 360-degree movements around the floor, and maybe moving backwards (babies have to move backwards before they can learn to go forwards). But this also means he can start exploring, so get down on your hands and knees and have a look around to see what a baby sees, what he can touch and what he can put into his mouth (for tips on baby-proofing your home, see pages 5–11).

I've taken many calls about babies swallowing coins, batteries, Lego and Scrabble pieces—just to name a few. But I'm never surprised, because babies are inquisitive and they do not know that Lego is not edible! All they do is react to objects and put them directly into their mouths—that's how they've learnt to feed themselves.

Daytime routine

Give your baby a drink of milk before he goes to sleep and when he wakes up in the morning. Then the day starts. The basic rule at six months—two hours up, then bed. So when the baby wakes up, get him up, give him a drink. Then feed, play, feed, play, and so on, for up to two hours, and put him back to bed. When your baby is about six or seven months, he may need a half-hour nap around 4 pm. But, if possible,

I would rather keep the baby up, as it's then easier for him to go down to sleep at night.

So, the morning session is again feed, play, feed, play. By this stage the baby is more active on the floor—definitely rolling, maybe commando crawling or wriggling backwards. Whatever activity he is doing, he needs to do a lot of it and you need to keep your eye on him because when he moves, he will move fast. Still continue to give him breast milk and/or formula.

If the baby is up at 7 am, offer him a drink of milk, then put him on the floor to play. After feeding him breakfast, put him back on the floor to play. When he starts grizzling, pick him up for a drink, then back down he goes onto the floor for more playtime.

Once he's been playing on the floor for about two hours, wrap him up or put him in a sleeping bag, and give him a drink of milk—I always give the baby a drink of milk before he goes to sleep and when he wakes up—then put him down for a sleep. Ideally he will sleep for 90 minutes to two hours in the morning and in the afternoon.

If your baby sleeps differently in the morning and in the afternoon, don't panic. Some babies sleep an hour in the morning then three hours in the afternoon, or an hour in the morning and an hour in the afternoon, with a half-hour nap in the late afternoon. So try not to expect your baby to sleep for a routine two hours and, when he doesn't, keep resettling him once he wakes up.

If he's waking up—pick him up, feed him, and start the feed, play, feed, play process again.

Afternoon/early evening routine

After the morning nap, get your baby up for a feed and then back to play. Once he's had some playtime it's into the highchair for lunch.

After lunch put him back down on the floor for feed, play, feed, play. It may be just a short play. When he has had enough time on the floor, pick him up for a feed, wrap him and then put him to bed.

The period between the lunchtime nap and bedtime can be hard because you're both tired—you've had a long day, the baby may be grizzly, and 7 pm seems hours away. Try to *avoid* going out in the car or going for a walk. Why? Because the baby will inevitably go to sleep but you want to keep him up so that, at the end of the day, he's tired and ready for bed.

So it's feed, play, feed, play, then dinnertime in the high-chair, followed by some play on the floor. Then it's bath time and into his onesie. Quietly read him a story in his room, then wrap him and put him into bed.

If your baby is not sleeping well at night or during the day, please read 'Passive settling' (see pages 181–89) because now is the time for you to get your baby into a nice bedtime routine.

Sleep

Congratulations on making the six-month mark! Seriously, as far as getting your baby to sleep goes, the hardest work is behind you. But if your child isn't sleeping that well at the moment, you may laugh when you read this. The good news is—this is the time when you can actually train your baby to sleep properly at night and for some good sessions during the morning and afternoon.

Wrapping and sleeping bags

There are a few changes to make now your baby is over six months old.

I've encouraged you to wrap your baby from birth using Cath's Wrap to make him feel nice and secure, calm and safe. By this stage your baby should be rolling quite capably on the floor, from back to front and front to back. Now that he is strong enough to roll well, you'll find that as soon as you put him into the cot he'll roll over onto his stomach to sleep.

When your baby was a newborn you followed the Sudden Unexpected Death in Infancy (SUDI) guidelines and put him to sleep on his back in the cot or bassinet. Now that he is older and stronger, he is capable of sleeping on his tummy all night. This makes a lot of parents anxious about the risk of SUDI, but you really can't police this developmental process without staying up all night, constantly turning the baby over from his tummy to his back. But there are some rules.

- There must be nothing in the cot with the baby—no blanket, cot bumper, comfort toys, pillow or doona. Nothing.
- The mattress must be firm and the right size for the cot—there must be no gaps between the mattress and the cot that the baby could slip into.
- A mattress protector and a clean fitted cot sheet are all you need to put on the mattress.

If your baby is not sleeping well overnight, or he's been sleeping in a bassinet beside your bed and you're transferring him to a cot, now is the time to practise passive settling (see pages 181–89). This is also the time to stop feeding your baby to sleep, remove the dummy (if he has one), and get your baby into a really good sleeping pattern, both day and night. You have been patient. Now go for it.

But before you start passive settling, there are a few things you should change.

- Remove Cath's Wrap so your baby is dressed only in a singlet and onesie. In winter, to keep his toes warm, put socks on his feet underneath the onesie.
- Dress him in a sleeping bag that leaves his arms out. There are so many fabulous sleeping bags on the market, so

choose one that suits the season—summer or winter—and make sure he has enough room to move.

- If your baby moves around so much in his sleep that his legs get tangled in the sleeping bag, waking him up, take off the bag and dress him in another layer of clothing to keep him warm.

- Most babies are comfortable in the sleeping bag and remain so for a couple of years. Just like the wrap, the sleeping bag tells the baby it's bedtime.

BBB routine

If you are still doing the BBB, now that your baby is more than six months old he will be well and truly ready to have a bath at 6.30 pm and go to bed at 7 pm. So that means following the bath with a breastfeed or a bottle, then off to bed in a sleeping bag. A dream feed at 10 pm (see page 164) is now in place of the original 10 pm bath and bottle that you started the day you came home from hospital.

I would expect a baby at this age to sleep until at least 4 am. When he wakes, give him a drink of breast milk or formula, then put him back to bed. He should sleep until 6 or 7 am.

You can continue the dream feed until your baby is 12 months, although some babies are not interested in the dream feed and totally refuse it. Either way, don't force him to take a bottle if he doesn't want it.

Crying after six months

By this age your baby should have established a pretty good sleep routine. But if he is consistently waking up after six months, you need to do something promptly. There are a few reasons why babies suddenly start waking up.

- He may be sick. With experience you'll come to recognise when your child is starting to come down with something—a couple of days before a child is actually ill his behaviour will usually change. If your child is clinging to you, crying, not eating or drinking, vomiting abnormally, has diarrhoea and/or feels hot, assume that he is unwell. It's safe to give him paracetamol every four to five hours according to his weight but you must follow the instructions on the packet.

- You are away on holidays. If you're away from home and your child is under 12 months, you will probably experience some sleepless nights. Babies are aware they're in a different environment and usually cry and have an unsettled night. While you're away, do what you can to get through the night.

- He is not getting enough playtime during the day. If your baby is sitting or lying flat and not getting enough exercise, he may wake up frequently during the night.

- He is teething.

- You use a dummy to resettle your baby.

- He is just in the habit of waking up and needs some passive settling to go back to sleep.

Passive settling

Do you want your baby to go back sleep by himself, but you don't have time for sleep school? This settling process is the only way to successfully get your baby back to sleep. It is safe, effective and efficient, and it works quickly. I practised passive settling with my own son when he was eight months old and waking every few hours after a bout of gastro.

I've also taught passive settling for well over 30 years, and the only babies who don't sleep properly are those who are picked up too early because their parents find it too hard to follow the process. I totally understand this, and I teach parents passive settling in their home because I know how hard it is to do it alone. I explain the process to both parents and make sure they understand it and agree to do it. Remember, it is actually better for the baby to sleep well and, of course, if he sleeps, you all sleep.

Overview

There are some strict rules, so read on . . .

Everyone has an opinion about this method—also called controlled crying—worrying that they're going to cause their child long-term harm but, believe me, a child waking up three to seven times a night will do far more harm to your parenting, and himself, than controlled crying. There are no published studies that show any evidence of physical or psychological harm resulting from controlled crying. More to the point, what is the effect of long-term sleep deprivation on a baby and his parents? It's not normal for a baby to wake every couple of hours, up to 10 times a night, and you need to get the baby to sleep for long periods overnight until he is old enough to sleep the night through. If you and your partner develop depression as a result of severe sleep deprivation—because being woken up frequently prevents you from going into a deep and healthy sleep—*that* will harm your baby.

So let's call it something else—*passive settling*. There, that sounds better, and we don't feel as if we're standing over our child 'controlling him' while he's 'crying his eyes out'.

Babies need to learn a skill before they can accomplish it, so if they're waking constantly overnight they need to learn to go back to sleep. The aim of passive settling is to teach the baby to go back to sleep by himself, but you must follow the procedure as I outline it in the pages that follow. Many parents have told me they tried passive settling many times but it never worked . . . but in my experience, if it didn't work it wasn't done properly!

To learn passive settling, your baby must:

- be over six months of age and/or weigh more than 8 kilograms

- show *no* signs of illness
- be in his own cot at home
- not be away from home within the next few weeks.

The method

1. Ensure your baby has had his dinner and bath by 6 pm. During the first session of passive settling try not to give him too much milk before bed in case he vomits, which will distress him and create more work for you. Offer lots of fluids during the day and a small drink of 50 ml before bed. If he's teething, give him the recommended dose of paracetamol per weight for his age. This not only ensures he is pain-free but also reassures you that he is not in pain.

2. Once your baby is ready for bed, dress him appropriately in a sleeping bag. Kiss him goodnight, tell him how much you love him, put him into bed and walk out the door. There should be no sheets, pillows or blankets in the cot. Leaving the baby crying in the cot is probably the hardest part. Remember, he is safe.

3. Then I suggest you fetch your phone and turn on the timer for two minutes. When your baby is crying, two minutes can seem like a very, very long time. It's best not to stand outside the door, listening to him crying. Do something to distract yourself—start emptying the dishwasher or make a cup of tea.

4. After the two minutes are up, go into the baby and reassure him, reciting the same mantra: 'Good night darling, time for bed. Good boy, I am here and I will be coming back. It's time to go to sleep. That's a good boy.'

5. Stay in the room, reassuring the baby, for only 15 to 20 seconds, then leave. If you stay there for a long time it will only stress both you and your baby. Many years ago we used to pick up the baby, hold him until he settled, then put him back in the cot. That process certainly took longer and only seemed to make the baby cry harder. Reassuring the baby in his cot is quicker and more efficient.

6. Once you have left the room, set the timer for four minutes and go through the same process.

7. Each time you leave the baby's room, increase the period between each visit according to this sequence—two-, four-, six-, eight-, 10- and 15-minute intervals. If the baby is still crying after 15 minutes, go in and settle him again. Then, if he is still crying after another 15 minutes, pick him up and feed him, then put him back to bed and he will sleep. You will achieve the same outcome.

In my experience I must say it's pretty rare for a baby to cry for 15 minutes. I find that between the four- and six-minute marks there tends to be a lull in the baby's crying, just for a few seconds. This is when you start to feel you've nearly achieved your goal.

All babies react differently to this process. Some take only half an hour to get it but others can seem to take hours. For passive settling to be successful, the baby must cry. His cry will intensify over the process and then as he settles the crying will settle down too. The aim for passive settling is for the baby to go to sleep.

When the baby stops crying and goes to sleep, you really won't believe the silence! High fives all round! When the baby is asleep and you have a monitor, you can leave him. Otherwise, check on him quietly. Look at him, but don't worry if he is up one end or other of the cot. Just leave him.

The next time the baby wakes up, wait for two minutes before going in to him. There is a slight chance that he may go back to sleep on his own. But if he hasn't after the two minutes, go in and start the process again. You do not need to give him paracetamol. I find during this part of the process the baby may settle quicker. High fives again!

Let me note here—you will find your first attempt at passive settling the most difficult: it will be emotionally demanding and take the longest time to achieve. But in reality your baby seems to learn to go back to sleep very quickly. If he wakes up again around 2 or 3 am, start the same settling process again, starting with two minutes, then four, and so on, as before.

Depending on the baby's age, if he goes to bed at 6 pm and sleeps through until 3 or 4 am, I would definitely feed the baby when he wakes. He will then go back to sleep for another few hours.

This method really works, so if you have a child who is waking constantly overnight, give it a go. Constantly patting and shushing a baby in a cot only distresses both the baby and the parents and, in my experience, doesn't work. I know the intervals between settling the baby can seem long, and you need support from your partner. If you 'break the rules' by stopping the process and feeding the baby, you will need to start again. So, once you start, be strong—and continue the whole process—until the baby is asleep.

The next day you need to continue passive settling for daytime sleeps. At sleep time, put the baby down into the cot and start the process again, leaving him to cry for two minutes, four minutes, six minutes, and so on. You will find that the baby very quickly gets the message and learns how to go to sleep.

Like many parents, I was sceptical about doing passive settling. Cath walked me through the process step by step, telling me it was going to be really hard and that I may feel like giving up (and I did, around about the six-minute mark). My baby was sleeping really well and for a decent number of hours, but she was really hard to get to sleep in the first place and settling her was taking longer and longer.

I know it sounds crazy but she was settling down to sleep so late at night that she slept in too late in the morning. I was bathing her at 8 pm and she wasn't settling until at least 9.30 pm. So eventually the night came when we had to bite the bullet and do passive settling. We bathed her at 6.30 pm, then I gave her a breastfeed and put her to bed by 7 pm. It was all over in about four minutes—she was asleep! I was astounded. I gave her a dream feed and she woke up at 4 am for a breastfeed and went back to sleep till 7 am—fabulous! She did this for four nights.

On the fifth night she really put up a fight, and that's when we really followed the whole passive settling routine. It took about 50 minutes but I now understand what Cath was saying: they have to increase their crying, then decrease it as they go to sleep. This is exactly what she did, and ever since then she has a breastfeed after her bath and a dream feed at 10 pm, then she wakes at 4 am for a breastfeed followed by a sleep until 8 am, when she is up for the day ahead. Even though she was a good sleeper, it's so much better now that I can put her down to bed while she's still awake and she goes straight to sleep on her own.

— LUCY

Important tips for success

1. It's vital that both you and your partner are committed to following the passive settling routine, because if one of you isn't determined, it won't work. Once you give in, you have to start again from scratch. But always remember the reward for sticking with it: you will sleep better, the baby will sleep better, and bingo, everyone feels a lot happier!

2. If you are still settling the baby with a dummy, you need to throw it out and follow the passive settling routine without it. Otherwise he will inevitably lose the dummy during the night and wake up crying.

3. If you are in the habit of feeding the baby to sleep—either by the breast or the bottle—again, you need to put the baby to bed awake. You'll find that he won't need to be fed to sleep once he's learnt to go to sleep by himself.

4. For some babies passive settling takes only a couple of days, but for others it can take up to a week. Either way, he won't be doing the hard crying you heard the first time you practised the passive settling routine. Instead, down the track, you might find that the baby wakes up at, say, 2 o'clock in the morning and just has a little bit of a grizzle for a couple of minutes. Before you've even got out of bed he's put himself back to sleep. That is the success of passive settling.

5. Remember that most babies have a little mantra they utter before they go to sleep. Some babies grizzle, some roll

around, sing or laugh, while others just have a cry and carry on. But they do go to sleep.

6. As I said earlier, some babies may vomit when crying hard, and that's why I really encourage you not to give your baby a big drink of milk before you put him to bed. If he has a good fluid intake during the day, a little sip of milk (50 ml) is quite enough before you put him to sleep.

7. If you feel you just can't handle it any longer and you want go in and pick up your baby . . . do it.

Not everyone agrees with controlled crying, but then not everyone has seen as many happy babies, and even happier and rested parents, as I have.

Listen to everything your child tells you. Even when he can't talk, listen to his cues. As a parent you know your child the best, and don't let any person tell you anything different. You are always the voice in your child's head.

10

Eight to ten months

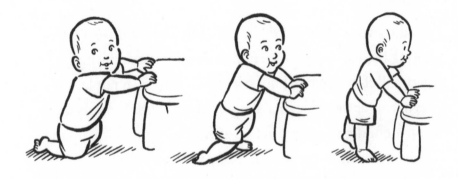

I'm loving food now, especially your lasagne. I love sleeping all night, and occasionally I'll wake up for a drink, but it's just a phase. I'm so busy now during the day, crawling and finding things to do like picking up coins from the floor—it was dangerous when I put one in my mouth. I'm so happy you are always close and keeping me safe. I sleep better during the day, too. I know I said 'da da da'. They're the easiest words for me to say. I could see you were proud of me! I love your cuddles and kisses.

Feeding your baby

Milk

By eight to 10 months your baby should be in a good routine with milk and food. Continue to breastfeed as often as you need to. Continue to offer milk first thing in the morning, before play, and before and after sleep. By this stage your child should be very active—definitely rolling, or even crawling.

Solids

Feeding your child solids in the early days creates lifelong eating habits, so try to keep mealtimes relaxed, positive and happy. Before feeding him, pop on his bib, then put him in a highchair at the table, making sure the harness is on securely. Some children are very active at this age and move around, so without his harness on it's easy for him to fall.

If he wants to eat from the spoon, let him do it and if he wants to eat finger food at the same time, that's fine too. Messy, but fine! He will be eating most of the foods you offer him. Now is a good time to offer him some milk in a sippy cup, even though he may not have the skill to put it up to his mouth and drink from it. Little steps, just take things slowly. Be patient.

Some babies are very sensitive to texture in their mouths and constantly gag when they're eating. If this is happening to your baby, just take it slowly. If you're in the habit of giving him a bowl of semi-puréed vegetables, don't suddenly introduce him to mashed food. You will have to slowly change the texture, which may take a few weeks. Encourage him to eat finger food.

From around eight months, a mixed diet is suitable. For breakfast each day you can mix small amounts of cow's milk along with yoghurt, cheese or custards into a breakfast cereal such as porridge. From nine months, introduce other cereals, such as Weet-Bix, with maybe some yoghurt and fruit.

Lunchtime can be some protein—either chicken or fish—followed by some fruit and yoghurt. And dinner can be vegetables with fish, chicken or meat. I usually offer morning and afternoon tea, maybe yoghurt, or some avocado. You will find out what your baby likes and dislikes very quickly.

It's okay if the baby doesn't have a huge variety in each meal as long as he has some chicken, fish or meat plus fruit, vegetables and, of course, his milk.

Development

Nine months

Gross motor	Fine motor
• Sits without support • Can get into a sitting position • Starting to pull to stand • Starting to crawl • Starting to stand holding on	• Starting to use a pincer grip—picking up small objects between his thumb and index finger

Social	Communication
• Exhibiting 'stranger danger' and separation anxiety and becoming clingier with familiar adults • Plays peekaboo • Starting to clap his hands • Recognises partly hidden objects and looks for objects that are hidden or dropped • Enjoys and demands attention and affection	• Babbling with consonants, such as 'baba', 'mama' • Starting to point • Copies sounds and gestures of others

Play

As far as play goes for a baby at this age, I'd be expecting him to be nearly crawling and then sitting up by himself. One really important thing to remember is that you do not sit your baby—he must crawl first, then learn to sit.

If you sit a baby at this age and surround him with lots of toys, he'll just keep sitting there. Even though he is capable of rolling, sitting or anything that stops your baby moving—a seat, a swing, or a walker—will prevent him from rolling and, in fact, have a negative impact on his progressive development. So don't let your extended family push you into sitting your baby, supported by pillows. Keep him flat on the floor and let him roll. He will gradually learn to get up on his hands and knees and start to rock. The next thing is learning to sit by himself. He may go backwards first, but eventually he will learn to crawl on his hands and knees.

By 12 months I expect babies to be cruising around the furniture, maybe standing or even walking, but if you interrupt his development by sitting him, walking will be delayed. This is when parents go to a professional to have their baby checked and are told that their baby isn't meeting his developmental milestones. Then the anxiety sets in. Specialists will examine the baby to see why he isn't moving.

The other long-term outcome of sitting a baby early is that he will do a 'bum shuffle' type of crawl. A lot of people think this looks really cute but in fact the proper way for a baby to crawl is on all fours! Babies who crawl on their hands and knees increase hand–eye coordination, fine motor skills, balance and special awareness. Skipping this important development stage may cause a baby to miss these developmental boosts.

So, this is when you don't listen to family or friends and keep your baby rolling on the floor and doing what his brain wants to do. It's beautiful to watch the purity of progressive development of a baby from newborn—helpless and dependent—to an active, potentially walking, talking personality at 12 months.

My baby didn't walk till he was 18 months old. The health professionals were worried and sent me to 'specialists' for my son to be checked. They found nothing wrong with him. I was beside myself with worry. It was not until I had my second baby and met Cath, who explained about the importance of floor play, that I understood where I went wrong with Sebastian. I had sat him on the floor, surrounded by hundreds of toys, since he was five months old. His sleeping overnight was terrible, but he was a happy baby during the day, just sitting!

It was a different story with baby number two. He rolled at 15 weeks, crawled at six months and was walking by 11 months. He never sat until he could sit himself. Lesson learnt.

— JANE

Daytime routine

Your baby is now waking up around 6 or 7 am—or even earlier—and has a drink from the breast or the bottle. Change his nappy, wash his hands and face, and also change his clothes, if necessary, then put him down on the floor to play until breakfast is ready. After breakfast, put him back on the floor to play or go out for a walk to the park.

Because your baby is now more active on the floor— commando crawling and maybe even crawling on hands and knees—all this activity needs to be supplemented with regular feeding. If he is grizzling, or if it's around two hours after he began playing on the floor, then give him some milk. Remember, when you are out and about with an eight-month-old, you can still do feed and play! After lunch, continue the feed, play, feed, play. I know I sound like a broken record but all this playtime and feeding is the *key* to your baby sleeping at night. It works!

Sleep

At eight months of age your baby can be in a settled sleeping routine. He is now capable of having a sleep in the morning, then another in the afternoon. Every child's sleep pattern is different. Your baby may sleep one hour in the morning and two in the afternoon and vice versa.

The basic rule at this age is two hours up, then a sleep. While some babies can cope with three hours of sleep, others will only stay asleep for one and a half hours. This really does vary across individual babies, so you need to respond to your own baby's needs. What works for your baby is right.

In the early eight-month days, he may need a little nap around 4 pm, just for half an hour, but I really would rather keep the baby up as then he's easier to go down to sleep at night.

I always give the baby a drink of milk before he goes to sleep and when he wakes up.

BBB routine

If you are still doing the BBB routine, then continue it. Your baby should be well over 8 kilograms by now, and be going to bed at 7 pm. That means giving him a bath at 6.30 pm, followed by a small play, a breastfeed or bottle and then reading him a book before bed.

I'd still offer a dream feed (see page 164) until he's 12 months, after which time I would remove this bottle feed. Some babies may still wake at the golden 4 am—don't try to fight it or try to resettle him. Simply feed him breast milk or a bottle then put him back to sleep until 6 or 7 am. You may find you get another three or so hours' sleep. Then the day starts.

Usually at this stage the baby, when placed into bed, spontaneously rolls over onto his tummy and sleeps all night. He doesn't need to be wrapped or in a sleeping bag. For bed, I would put his onesie on and, if necessary during winter, a long-sleeved singlet and socks under his onesie to keep his toes warm. We adults are so used to having pillows, doonas and lots of clothes on at night and we expect a baby needs and wants them, too. But if you have dressed him warmly he is quite okay.

Remember, there should be absolutely nothing in his cot—no bumper, no toys, nothing. Just a good mattress and a clean fitted sheet. Babies move around a lot in the cot during the night, and sometimes they sit up and even stand. A lot of mums think that sleeping bags are a 'sleeping tool' to help the baby go to sleep. I find them the opposite in some cases. When babies reach this age of eight months and older they tend to be really active in bed overnight. You will be surprised; if you put your baby down and then watch him on the monitor you will see how much he moves around the cot. All around, up and down. He may sit up, then lay back down.

Why your baby's sleeping pattern might change

If there's any change in your baby's sleeping pattern it's usually due to one of the following:

- illness
- travel
- dummy (or pacifier)
- change of environment.

To get sleeping back on track, try the passive settling technique again (see pages 181–89), but remember:

- if he's been sick, the baby needs to be well and recovered
- you need to be in your own home, and not about to go away
- you need to throw the dummy out (which is usually more stressful for the parents than the baby).

Travelling

Travelling with children can be a nightmare but, if you're lucky, it can also be seamless. What you can depend on is that when you get onto the plane, everyone will stare at you, with a look on their faces that says, 'Please don't sit next to me.' You immediately regret every time you stared at new parents with a baby, struggling into the plane seats next to you.

As the plane takes off and lands, a baby needs to suck either on the breast or on a bottle to equalise the pressure on his eardrums. If your baby has a cold while you are travelling, he will scream when the plane starts to descend. Always have paracetamol on hand in case your baby has ear pain.

Once you reach your destination, you may wonder why on earth you left home—it is such a drama to get everything packed for a holiday and then the baby doesn't sleep in the unfamiliar environment . . . But you can't stay home forever.

When to leave work, and when to return

I know from all my experience that it's better for both mother and baby for the pregnant mum to finish work earlier rather than later, but a lot of women say to me, 'I only have an office job, sitting at a desk.' They still have to get out of bed, get into the office and work all day, then go home. By the time most women get close to finishing work, around 36 or 37 weeks, they are completely over being pregnant and feeling very uncomfortable and tired.

When you go on maternity leave, enjoy time off before your baby is born. You will never have this break again, so relish it. I encourage you to have a rest after lunch each day. With so many wonderful shows now streaming on television, and podcasts to listen to, you can be entertained while you rest. Some silence, or reading a book, is also therapeutic. When you rest, your baby rests, too.

Going back to work is always a challenging issue for women. The time to do so is when *you* are ready—when you need to start earning money again, or when you miss your work and/or can't afford to interrupt your career path. For women who don't find being at home with a baby full-time fulfilling, balancing part-time work and parenting is ideal. Deciding when, or even if, to go back to work is no one's business but your own.

> I have had three children. I love them but I don't love being a stay-at-home mum. It just isn't for me. I went back to work full-time when each child was six months old. They went into childcare and my parents helped too. I was, and still am, a better and happier mum for returning to work. I know it's not for everyone but it is for me. I have had plenty of

comments (mostly negative), like, 'How could you leave your baby?' When I went back to work after my first child turned six months old, I was very upset by people's comments, but I know I am a good and happy mum and my children are happy and healthy.

— STEPHANIE

Childcare

Choosing childcare is really difficult. I was fortunate my son Lachlan was cared for by his grandparents while he was young, as it made going back to work a lot easier for me. In the years he spent with my mum and dad, he learnt so much, and he went on more trains, trams and buses that I ever would have taken him on. Now that he's an adult he has wonderful memories of his grandparents caring for him.

When Lachlan was three, I used the council-run family day care. It was tremendous, and I was very lucky that some wonderful women cared for him within a home environment.

It certainly is very stressful having a child in care while you're working—well, I found it stressful. But after a long day at work I loved arriving home, hopping out of my work clothes, cooking dinner and hearing about my son's day. I love being a mum.

These days there are lots of childcare options to choose from.

- Before your child is born, investigate childcare centres near your home or work. Most centres have long waiting lists.
- Also check out family day care—a home-based childcare service, run by local councils.
- If you can afford it, you can share a nanny with another mum or family.
- You can share the care with your partner, and/or ask grandparents to help on certain days.

Choosing childcare—what matters most

Whatever childcare option you choose, you should feel happy about the people who are caring for your child. Before you employ a nanny in your home, ask for references. Ideally, meet the person who wrote the reference in person. You are leaving your precious child with someone you may know nothing about.

If you have certain ways of doing things with your child, tell the people who are caring for him. For example, tell your nanny how your child's day runs; don't let him or her run your child's day.

Always make sure the people who are caring for your children have had a Working With Children Check (WWCC), which includes a National Police Check. This is a requirement Australia-wide, but a childcare worker cannot move to another state and use their original certified documents—they will need a WWCC for the state in which they're currently working.

Look after yourself. Eat well, drink plenty of water and have some rest during the day—even if it's a ten-minute nap while your baby sleeps. Being a parent means you are always thinking about the needs of your baby, but your baby needs you to be well and happy.

11

Ten to twelve months

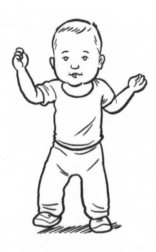

I'm so excited I'm nearly one. I can hear you organising my birthday party. How good is life now. I love making lots of noise. Thank you for the blocks, they are so much fun to bang together. I'll be able to see my friends at childcare now you are back at work. How clever am I . . . taking five steps today all by myself. I'm a bit nervous and had a few spills but I love that you stay with me to keep me safe and confident. I love you.

Feeding your baby

Milk

Coming up to 12 months, there are a lot of changes taking place. By this stage your baby will still be drinking breast milk and/or formula. As he approaches 11 and a half months, you can transition him from formula to full cream cow's milk.

If your baby hasn't had any formula, and only water from a sippy cup, offer him at least three cups of milk a day. By this stage, he would have had cow's milk on his cereal in the morning along with yoghurt, cheese, custard and maybe even some ice cream during the day.

If he is on formula, change over to full cream cow's milk— but do it slowly. You need to give your baby full cream cow's milk in small amounts over a few weeks so the baby tolerates it and most importantly becomes accustomed to the taste. We want him to like milk, so we need to introduce it slowly. If you give him a full glass of full cream milk his gut may not tolerate it and he may have diarrhoea. To transition the baby to full cream cow's milk properly, follow the sequence described below.

How to transition from formula to full cream cow's milk
Offer your baby his drink in a sippy cup, but adjust the ratio of formula to cow's milk in the following way. If at any time the baby has diarrhoea, vomiting or a rash or refuses the milk,

go back a step and offer him less cow's milk for four days, then start again.

1. Offer him 100 ml of formula and 20 ml of cow's milk.
2. Two days later, offer 80 ml of formula and 40 ml of cow's milk.
3. Two days later, offer 60 ml of formula and 60 ml of cow's milk.
4. Two days later, offer 40 ml of formula and 80 ml of cow's milk.
5. Two days later, offer 20 ml of formula and 100 ml of cow's milk.
6. Two days later, offer the baby full cow's milk.

In this way you gradually change the formula over to cow's milk, giving him a chance to adjust to this new taste. Imagine if I told you to drink a bottle of formula—you wouldn't instantly like the taste and the texture. As long as you change over from formula gradually, your baby will be happy to drink cow's milk.

Continue to give him cow's milk three times a day, plus cheese, plus custard.

How to transition from full breast milk to full cream cow's milk

The same rules apply to transitioning from breast milk to full cream cow's milk. If your baby reacts by vomiting, or has diarrhoea or a rash, the same rules apply—go back a step and offer him less cow's milk for four days, then start again, taking it very slowly. If he hasn't had any formula in the previous 12 months, there is no need to offer him any.

1. Offer him a sippy cup of 100 ml of water and 20 ml of cow's milk.
2. Two days later, offer 80 ml of water and 40 ml of cow's milk.
3. Two days later, offer 60 ml of water and 60 ml of cow's milk.
4. Two days later, offer 40 ml of water and 80ml of cow's milk.
5. Two days later, offer 20 ml of water and 100 ml of cow's milk.
6. Two days later, the baby is ready to take full cow's milk.

The beauty of slowly transitioning a baby from breast milk to cow's milk is that he will like cow's milk, and we want him to drink adequate amounts in these early years. Of course, you can continue to breastfeed your baby as well as give him cow's milk.

Replacing the bottle with a sippy cup

At around 10 months offer water in a sippy cup after meals. Around 12 months is a good time to stop giving your baby a bottle and replace it with a sippy cup.

I've always put a circle around 12 months on the calendar for lots of 'growing up' changes for the baby—one of them being removing the bottle. I find that if you don't remove the bottle at 12 months, you'll still be giving the baby a bottle at two years, three years, even four years of age. The baby doesn't need a bottle—a sippy cup or a cup with a straw is adequate.

Lots of parents don't want to take the bottle away from the baby, thinking it's a comfort and that the baby loves having it. It's not the end of the world if the baby does continue with the bottle, but if he takes a bottle to bed and you don't clean his teeth before he goes to sleep, the sugar in the milk can potentially damage his gums and milk teeth.

Solids

As your baby moves towards 12 months of age, increase the range and quantity of foods you offer him. At the end of his first year, he should be consuming a wide variety of family foods, having progressed from purées or mash to foods that are chopped into small pieces. He should be offered most of what the rest of the family is eating, having tried food that needs chewing, such as meat and chicken. By now he will have been offered all fruit and all vegetables.

By 12 months your child can eat everyday family foods *unless* there are allergies (see 'Introducing foods that may cause allergies', pages 171–73). Ensure your child has plenty of fruit, vegetables and beans along with cereals, rice, pasta, noodles and other grains.

It's really important to avoid making dinnertime anxiety time. I know I've said it before, but put the baby in the highchair for meals. Always put his harness on. Offer him his meal and, when he's finished eating, take him out of the highchair. By doing things such as consistently using his harness, you're helping your child to understand that sitting and eating means mealtime. Of course, there are always exceptions to the rule—some children totally refuse to eat solids by 10 to 12 months, causing their parents a lot of anxiety that is then transferred to the baby.

A child who refuses food

If your child refuses food, my advice is not to dance around him or put the television on to distract him in order to ensure he eats. These are not good practices. Your child is not going to starve. Children are very sensible and sensitive, and they know when they need to eat and what they want to eat. As I've said before, your baby does not need gourmet food. What he does need is good clean food, with you sitting quietly next to him—either feeding him with a spoon or letting him eat with his fingers. He will learn table manners as he gets older and his brain develops, so don't get distressed if mealtimes are messy.

Development

Twelve months

Gross motor	Fine motor
• Starting to cruise around furniture • Starting to stand unassisted • May take first steps	• Bangs two objects together • Puts things in a container and can take things out of a container • Pokes with his index finger

Social	Communication
• Stronger stranger danger • Has favourite things and people • Puts out an arm or leg to help with dressing • Shows needs and wants in ways other than crying	• Starting to use simple gestures, such as shaking head for 'no', or waving goodbye • Making sounds with changes of tone • Saying 'mama' and 'dada' with more meaning • Starting to imitate sounds said to him • Starting to understand simple commands • Starting to understand the meaning of 'no'

Play

At 10 to 12 months of age your baby is a delight to play with. He is interactive and he loves games! Babies have an insatiable appetite for fun.

Activities babies love at this age

Bedtime stories are a must—babies love stories and often have a favourite book. Believe me, you will read it to him over and over and over again, and he will re-enact and remember parts of the story. Small books with just one object on a page—such as 'A for Apple', 'B for Bottle', 'C for Cat'—are really good books to start with. They are simple. Remember that your child does not have a good concentration level at this age.

He will love blocks and building towers and knocking them down, because developmentally he's crawling and sitting by himself by this stage. He also loves playing peekaboo and any games that provide fun.

Remember that you don't have to keep on playing the *same* game with your baby. It's like tickling a baby. It can be very distressing for him to be tickled constantly. While a few tickles are cute, any more is annoying. If you see friends or family constantly tickling your baby and you feel uncomfortable about it, remember you are your baby's voice and say, 'How about just a few tickles, then change the game—that's what the baby likes.' You can go 'kitchy, kitchy, koo', but when you keep doing that to a baby he really does tire of it and will disengage with you. When he turns away or begins to whinge, that's the sign he wants to stop that game. So keep games quick, short and varied.

Babies at this age love dancing, which usually consists of them standing with you holding them under their armpits, then bending their knees and moving with the music.

A safety warning here—never swing or pull your baby up by the hands. This applies to all children up to the age of five years. This can cause dislocation of the wrist and elbows very easily and causes severe pain to the baby. The baby would need to have the elbow or wrist popped back in by a doctor. It is really important you tell members of the family and talk up if you see the baby being swung around by his hands during playtime. Remember you are his voice.

Babies also love putting toys in boxes and taking them out again. But nothing is more exciting for them than extracting a thousand tissues from a tissue box. The problem with this game is that you have to pick up all the tissues! If you can be bothered, buy some cheap handkerchiefs and put them in an empty tissue box. Your baby can pull them out and you can put them back in again, rather than have tissues strewn all over the house.

Climbing

Some children climb—and they start early. They climb on chairs, onto the table, the bed, couches—in fact, they climb on everything. And that's just inside the house. Outside, there are climbing structures specially designed for children in parks and playgrounds. If you have a 'climber', you will spend the first five years of your child's life in parks and play-grounds. It's not only boys. Some girls are amazing climbers, too, and it's not uncommon to find them on the table, dancing and jumping!

Children climb for fun, to explore, to access toys and to see life from a different perspective. Children at this age are hardwired to climb and have no sense of danger or fear. This, of course, brings parents unending fear, but as long as you stay close, keep the area safe and your eyes on them, climbing is fine; in fact, it is an important learning skill required for healthy and progressive development and education. It starts at birth, with your baby moving his head from side to side when doing tummy time, learning to lift his head and shoulders from the ground to look up and around. Once he learns to roll from back to front, then from front to back, he embarks on the progressive movement that Mother Nature has designed for him.

But before he can contemplate climbing, your baby needs to achieve certain developmental skills. He needs to move backwards before he goes forwards, so in the early days you may find him underneath the couch with his head poking out.

Your baby requires hundreds of hours of crawling on his hands and knees before he can lift himself up and cruise along the furniture. Once cruising, he will gain confidence and momentum and then, one day, he will stand alone. Legs apart, arms outstretched—a picture of perfect balance.

Once he is confident standing, he begins making those exciting steps forward, literally one step at a time. There will be lots of tumbles and falls along the way but it's best to allow your baby to learn at his own pace rather than give him objects, such as trolleys, to push. Your baby requires all these skills in order to satisfy his curiosity by climbing, exploring and viewing the world.

> By the time my daughter was 10 months old, she could stand alone for seconds at a time and crawl up stairs, faultlessly, squealing with excitement all the way. It wasn't long before she started climbing, and it then became obvious that we'd have to remove the gates at the top and bottom of the stairs or risk her having a terrible accident. She was just one of those really active, curious and adventurous babies, and you had to keep her in your line of sight all the time.
>
> — ALICE

Sleep

In the daytime

Sleep for babies at this age should stay much the same until after 12 months. I would expect a baby to be up for two hours after breakfast and play, then back down to sleep after two hours. Of course, some babies will be capable of staying up for three hours while others will only manage staying awake for one and a half hours. So it's up to you how your baby is managing being awake and playing. Don't stick to rigid routines by the clock, as this will only stress you—and your baby. If you go out some days and the baby has his nap while you are driving . . . that's okay. The main aim is that you are all happy and well.

At night

Ideally, by this age your baby is sleeping well overnight—and I mean from 6 pm to 6 am. If you have a 10- to 12-month-old baby who is waking frequently, or sleeping with you in your bed (at some point most of us sleep with our children), I suggest this is the time to do something about it . . . before you are all sleep deprived. The best, easiest and most effective way to get a child this age back to sleep is by passive settling (see pages 181–89).

BBB routine

By this age the BBB routine is pretty well set in concrete.

After dinner, around 5.30 pm, the baby has his last drink of milk, then you clean his teeth, bath him, read him a few stories and put him to bed for the night.

Occasionally, some babies still have the dream feed (see pages 164), but if a baby's weight is satisfactory and he is having enough milk during the day, this is not necessary.

So the BBB routine comes to an end. It started right back on the very first night you came home from hospital and you (or your partner) bathed your new baby at 10 pm. I hope you have enjoyed the time spent with your baby in the first 12 months and the closeness, bonding and love you have shared with your little baby in his first year.

The bath routine continues through childhood. But nothing will be as special as those first 12 months of bathing, wrapping your little baby, breastfeeding him or giving him a nice bottle of milk and putting him to bed safely. These are the stories you will tell him as he gets older, and at his 21st. Hopefully they will encourage him to do exactly the same things when he becomes a parent.

Shoes

Most children usually walk around the age of 12 months. They start by cruising around the furniture, then standing, then walking. For babies learning to walk, it's always best to let them walk with bare feet, then progress to softer shoes, and, finally, well-fitted shoes once they have been walking for a few months. You can buy soft shoes with some traction underneath the sole.

Always have your child's first shoes fitted by an experienced shoe fitter in a major department store. The shoe should be light and flexible—lace-up shoes are recommended. Children at this age grow quickly, so you don't need the most expensive shoes in the store. But, most importantly, they must fit the child properly.

Thumb sucking and dummies

Thumb sucking is normal for some babies. Not all children suck their thumb but the ones who do so usually do it for comfort. It makes them feel happy and secure, and it's harmless.

Young children may also suck to soothe themselves and help them fall asleep. Most parents worry about the effect on their teeth, and it can cause some problems if a child sucks very hard with his thumb on his palate. After the permanent teeth come in there can be problems with growth of the mouth and alignment of the teeth.

Dummies have the same effect as thumbs but are easy to throw away. I find the dummy is actually a problem for the *parents* to give up, as they can come to rely on it and later have an issue with letting it go. A child will continue to suck a dummy as long as parents continue to give it to them and even attach it to them. My advice would be to remove the dummy at six months. If I do passive settling, I remove the dummy at the same time. They may not be that clean anyway and may cause ear and throat infections.

Television, tablets and smart phones

In an era when technology has such an important place in our lives—from the internet and television to tablets and smart phones, streaming music and television services—we need to address how we manage this technology with our children. It amazes me how infants as young as 12 months can swipe a smart phone open, put in the code and go to their favourite app!

As clever as these devices are, it's risky to put them into our children's hands. I believe that anything in moderation is fine, but smart phones and tablets are being used as parenting tools. I grew up with television; we watched our shows after school and it was fun but, in hindsight, some of the shows were probably violent. These days, the information you can access online is really disturbing, especially for children. The good news is that there are phone locks and parental access tools that can limit a child's access to this content.

Of course, these devices have a place in our lives; there is nothing better than looking at movies on your tablet, computer or phone when you want to relax or when you're travelling. But these gadgets are addictive, and they should not be used as babysitters or as a substitute for parenting.

The importance of setting limits

It takes a lot of boundary setting to ensure a child has a limited time on a smart phone or tablet, because they can scream. And they can scream *really* loud when they want something.

As parents, we don't want to hear our children upset or screaming, and so often we give in. But by giving in, we give them what they want. That is the easy way out. It's okay to limit access and say: '"No" means "no"—it doesn't mean keep asking me until I say "yes".' Learning these rules as a young child is so important. These boundaries will become set in stone in his head and, when he is a teenager, they will still apply.

If your child screams and throws a tantrum to get your smart phone or tablet, there are three things you can do: you can give it to him instantly, let him scream or distract him, by giving him something else. I encourage distraction because children at this age do not have the developmental capacity to understand what they are consuming at such a young age.

Disciplining your child

Hitting children as 'discipline'—a bad idea!

When you have a child, you are tired and busy. Often your reaction to your child can make you feel guilty and regretful. There isn't a single parent who doesn't feel some confusion when it comes to dealing with challenging child behaviour. Fifty to 60 years ago, children were smacked not only by their parents but also routinely by their teachers at school.

Hitting a child is often driven by your anger and frustration. It doesn't teach a child tolerance or how to cope with a challenging situation later in life. If you hit a child when you're frustrated, I can tell you that when they go to school and feel frustrated themselves, the first thing they'll do is hit. That's not socially acceptable—you'll find your child will have issues later on, not only at school, but for the rest of his life.

Praise good behaviour—and ignore bad behaviour

Some parents don't want to discipline their child at all, as they want to avoid any conflict; they don't want their child to be annoyed or angry at them. We need to find a balance between hitting a child and letting him get away with any sort of behaviour that may harm him or others. My mantra is 'praise good behaviour and ignore bad behaviour'. Ensure that your child is safe when you are ignoring his behaviour.

You must remember the age of the child, and their developmental capacity, when you are putting boundaries on their behaviour. A child of 10 to 12 months has no idea of right or wrong, so trying to reason with him when he's having a tantrum is a battle *no one* will win. Parents require a lot of patience, especially when your child is this age. Children usually 'settle down' at some level when they are about four years of age—that's the good news! The bad news is that being a parent requires consistent hard work—but if you work at it during the early years, believe me, the reward is a sensible and hopefully settled teenager.

A child goes through different developmental milestones—their brain develops at a rate that is capable of coping with the demands and stresses of particular ages. So just as a child of 12 months cannot drive a car—he is developmentally incapable of having the necessary skills to understand the complexities required for that set of skills—we must be mindful that a child of 10 to 12 months has limited capabilities when it comes to decision-making, behaviour and the capacity to play with another child. We parents are the teachers, the guides. Our voices and our behaviour provide the models for how our children are going to develop and see the world. So it's up to us to play an important and consistent role in the development of our children's early social and emotional skills.

Just by your tone of voice or facial expression, your newborn baby understands, and is sensitive to, how you are reacting to him. So talk to your baby, talk to your three-month-old, four-month-old, ten-month-old, one-year-old—just talk, talk, talk. Even though you want to say, 'I've had a really bad day and I am over this parenting gig', talk to him in a positive and loving way. I understand it's hard—I've been there, done that, got the t-shirt! I put some words and phrases on the fridge door and when I felt tired and frustrated, I'd look at those words and use them in a positive tone. Often I'd be saying things such as 'What a good job you're doing' rather than 'Stop doing that'. Babies learn from your tone of voice and facial expressions—so positive parenting and tone of voice is *everything* in the early days.

Being a good parent doesn't require a specialised qualification in early development. But being well informed can help you be more effective in ensuring your child enjoys the appropriate experiences he needs in order to reach his potential. You need to inform yourself about the developmental capacities of your child. This will help you parent positively and certainly help you interact with your child in a happier and more positive way.

If you don't understand your child's developmental stages, you might expect even a 10- to 12-month-old baby to be capable of understanding complex issues and, when he doesn't meet your expectations, become impatient and angry with him, then discipline him inappropriately. Your child doesn't know what he has done wrong. *It's all about patience.*

Every child is his own person. He is no one else. He has the right to be loved and cared for as he moves, explores and learns about this complex world we live in. As parents we have to be there to hold his hand, protect him, teach him all about life. And parenting is one of the most rewarding jobs in the world.

Sample feeding chart

Use this chart to keep track of your child's initial reactions to solids as you introduce each new food. See 'Introducing foods that may cause allergies', pages 171–73.

Date given	Eggs	Nuts	Dairy	Fish	Comments

SAMPLE FEEDING CHART

Date given	Poultry	Meat	Fruit	Vegetables	Comments

Percentile growth charts

Boys length-for-age percentiles

Birth to 12 months

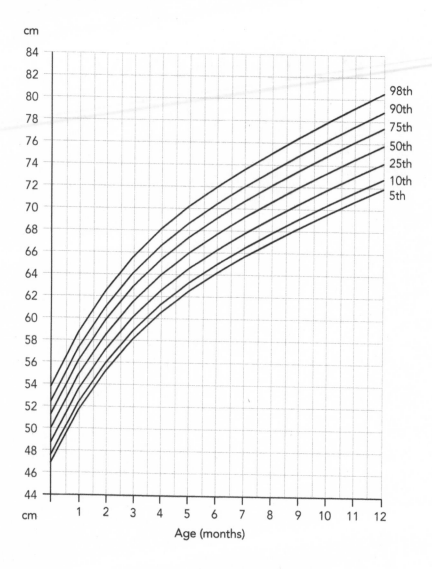

Source: World Health Organisation Child Growth Standards http://www.who.int/childgrowth/en

Girls length-for-age percentiles

Birth to 12 months

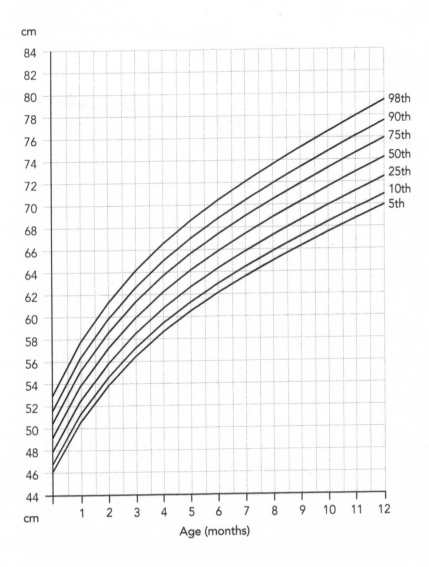

cm

84
82
80 — 98th
78 — 90th
76 — 75th
74 — 50th
72 — 25th
70 — 10th
5th
68
66
64
62
60
58
56
54
52
50
48
46
44
cm

Age (months)

Source: World Health Organisation Child Growth Standards http://www.who.int/childgrowth/en

233

Boys weight-for-age percentiles

Birth to 12 months

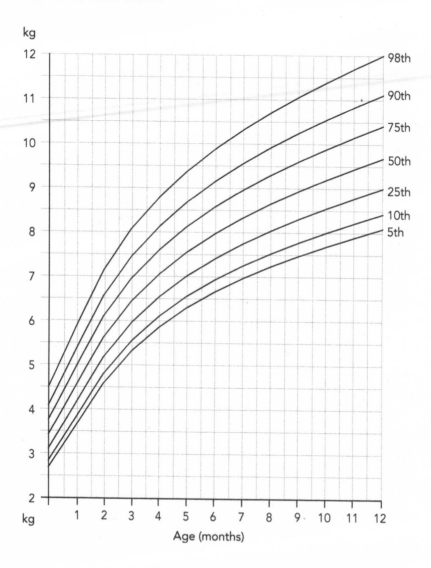

Source: World Health Organisation Child Growth Standards http://www.who.int/childgrowth/en

Girls weight-for-age percentiles

Birth to 12 months

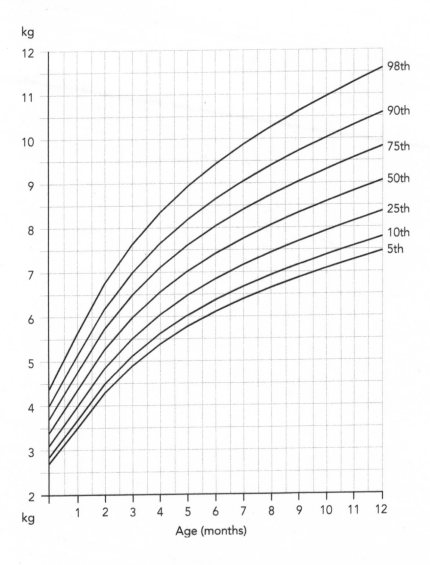

Age (months)

Source: World Health Organisation Child Growth Standards http://www.who.int/childgrowth/en

Boys head circumference-for-age percentiles

Birth to 12 months

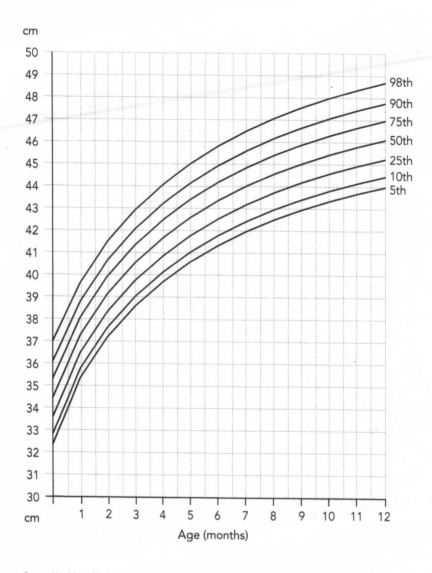

Source: World Health Organisation Child Growth Standards http://www.who.int/childgrowth/en

Girls head circumference-for-age percentiles

Birth to 12 months

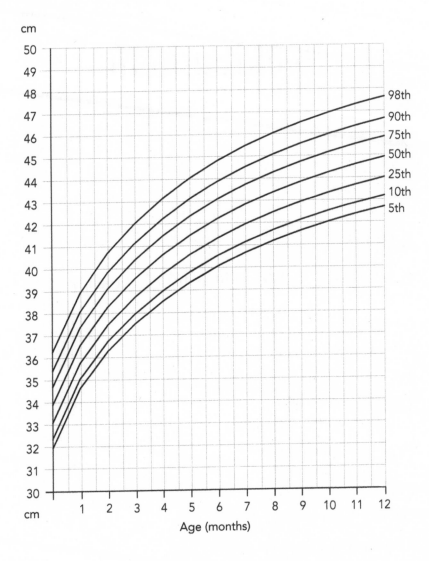

cm

Age (months)

Source: World Health Organisation Child Growth Standards http://www.who.int/childgrowth/en

Seeking help

SANDS

For miscarriage, stillbirth and newborn death support

National office
Level 2b, 818 Whitehorse Road,
Box Hill, Victoria, 3128
Tel: (03) 9895 8700
Email: support@sands.org.au
Web: www.sands.org.au

Queensland
Tel: (07) 3254 3422
Email: admin@sandsqld.com
Web: www.sandsqld.org.au

South Australia
Tel: 0417 681 642
Email: info@sandssa.org.au
Web: www.sandssa.org.au

Tasmania
Tel: 0415 127 464
Email: tasmania@sands.org.au
Web: www.sandstas.org.au

Victoria
Tel: (03) 9874 5400
Email: victoria@sands.org.au
Web: www.sandsvic.org.au

Western Australia
Tel: 0424 340 115
Email: adminwa@sands.org.au
Web: www.sandswa.org.au

Parenting helplines

Grandcare (information service for grandparents)
Tel: 1800 008 323

Karitane Careline
Tel: 1300 227 464

Maternal and Child Health Line
Tel: 13 22 29

Ngala Helpline
Tel: 1800 111 546 (STD callers) or (08) 9368 9368

Parentline ACT
Tel: (02) 6287 3833

Parentline NSW
Tel: 1300 1300 52

Parentline Queensland and Northern Territory
Tel: 1300 301 300

Parent Helpline South Australia
Tel: 1300 364 100

Parentline Tasmania
Tel: 1300 808 178

Parentline Victoria
Tel: 13 22 89

Parenting WA Line
Tel: 1800 654 432 (STD callers) or (08) 6279 1200

13 HEALTH
Web: www.health.qld.gov.au/13health/
Tel: 13 43 25 84

Tresillian Parent Helpline
Tel: 1300 272 736 or 1300 2 Parent

General helplines

Alcohol Drug Information Service (ADIS)
Tel: 1800 422 599, (02) 9361 8000 (Sydney metro)

Child Care Access Hotline
Tel: 1800 670 305 or 133 677
(TTY service for people with a hearing/speech impairment)

Child Wise National Child Abuse Helpline
Tel: 1800 99 10 99

Family Relationship Advice Line
Tel: 1800 050 321

Health Direct Australia (not available in Victoria or Queensland)
Tel: 1800 022 222

Kids Helpline
Tel: 1800 55 1800

Lifeline
Tel: 13 11 14

Medicare
Tel: 132 011

Mensline Australia (support and referral to specialist men's services)
Tel: 1300 78 99 78

National Breastfeeding Helpline
Tel: 1800 MUM 2 MUM or 1800 686 268

National Poisons Information Centre
Tel: 13 11 26

National Sexual Assault, Domestic Family Violence Counselling Service
Tel: 1800 RESPECT or 1800 737 732

Playgroup Australia
Tel: 1800 171 882

Sane Australia Helpline
Tel: 1800 187 263

Acknowledgements

I could not have finished this book without the love and support of my darling son Lachlan and his wonderful fiancée Bella. They looked after me and were my biggest cheer squad. Thank you Lach and Bella, this book is dedicated to you both with all my love. It's an honor to be your mum, Lach, I am so proud of you and love you very much.

I was still recovering from having written one book when Claire Kingston from Allen and Unwin asked me to write a second. Thanks Claire for your belief in my parenting methods—because of your support many parents are sleeping better overnight and I have a voice in the wider community supporting women in pregnancy and parenting. Thank you also to Kelly Fagan and Rebecca Allen from A&U for all your wonderful help, support and direction.

Sarah Baker was the main editor on this book as she was on *The First Six Weeks* and without her incredible magic, amazing support and understanding of my parenting methods, this book would make no sense. Sarah, thank you for your calm and methodical approach. You are a lifesaver and you will forever be a huge part of my books. Thank you.

To Joseph Farago, Lina and Hezi Leibovich, Al Grigor and Lara Fekete—my amazing friends, thank you so much for your love and support over the past few years. I have a small group of close friends who have been a great support to me, thank you Ky, Gwen, Brydie, Emily, Brooke, Tony, Dave, Kim and Clare.

Thanks to my fellow professionals Elise Swallow, Nichols Pakkiam, Brendan Chan, Ben Gold for your contribution to the book.

Index